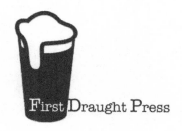
First Draught Press

The ICU Survival Book

William Owens, MD

First Draught Press
MMXXII

Medicine is an ever-changing discipline, and the subject matter of this book is no exception. While the author has done his best to ensure that this book reflects contemporary evidence-based practice, new developments in the field may supersede the material published here. Only properly trained and licensed practitioners should provide medical care to patients. Nothing in this book should be construed as advice regarding the care of a specific patient or group.

Cover Design by Lorien Owens

Published by First Draught Press
Columbia, SC

ISBN 978-0-9852965-7-5

Printed in the United States of America

Lorien has been my wife, my fellow adventurer, and my editor-in-chief for nearly twenty years. I am grateful for everything she did to push me to write this book—I can honestly say that it would not have happened without her.

William, Zach, and Amelia—I am proud to dedicate this book to you. Being your dad is my most important job.

TABLE OF CONTENTS

IT WAS A DARK AND STORMY NIGHT...

The start of many a dramatic story, and the scene of many of an intern's* greatest fears. Insert "in the ICU" to the end of the phrase, and it conjures visions of ventilator alarms, unstable dysrhythmias, and lots of blood.

The reality is that your ICU rotation is more likely to seem like a long march through the mountains. There will be hard times, easier times, and unforeseen events. The only thing that's consistent is that it's *work.* Yes, I know that residency in general is tough. Yes, I know that the ward services also have a lot of patients and that their residents have a lot to do. But I also know that there's something about the ICU that is simultaneously intimidating and exhilarating. The key, and the goal of this book, is to make it more of the latter than the former.

Let's start with something that seems basic, but is important: what, exactly, is an ICU?

The ICU is a place for the treatment of actual or impending organ system failure. It is a place for close physiological monitoring and for intervening when things go awry, and it is a place for the application of advanced technology that can't be done elsewhere in the hospital.

---

* At this point, you may be thinking, "Wait a minute! I'm not an intern. I'm a medical student/nursing student/PA/NP! Did I buy the wrong book?" Relax. Healthcare has become increasingly interdisciplinary over the last few years, and that's been a good thing. "Intern" is an older term for a PGY-1 medical resident, but in this book it's shorthand for anyone who is relatively new to Critical Care Medicine.

1

In order to make that happen, then, the ICU needs specialized staff who are capable of monitoring and providing care to critically ill and injured patients. Nurses typically have two patients at a time, or maybe just one if he's extra-complicated. Respiratory therapists who are trained in the management of mechanical ventilators are part of the staff, as are critical care PharmDs, critical care nutritionists, and specialist physical therapists. Physicians and Advanced Practice Providers round on the unit and direct the treatment plan.

And then there's **you**.

As a newcomer, the ICU may appear overwhelming. There's just so much to learn! How can you possibly learn everything there is to know to take care of critically ill patients in such a short time? After all, your rotation is only a month!

Here's the truth. Pay attention:

1. No one expects you to know everything. You're here to learn.
2. No one will let you do anything to hurt a patient. The system is set up for safety. That's why there are experienced ICU nurses, a PharmD, a respiratory therapist, an ICU fellow, and an ICU attending also paying attention.
3. There is only one skill that is essential to becoming a successful clinician, and it's the one thing you need to focus on developing during your time in the ICU.

That skill? It's not knowing how to manage a ventilator, or how to titrate vasopressors, or how to decipher an ABG. It's much simpler, and yet much more difficult. **It's the ability to differentiate sick from not sick.**

Why is that tough? It's because we're not talking about the extremes. A patient on a ventilator, multiple vasopressor infusions, and in a coma? Easy. Sick. Another patient who walked into the ED, has normal vital signs, and is there for a cut on her finger? Easy. Not sick.

That's not the challenge. The challenge is recognizing that the man with low back pain and dizziness has an aortic aneurysm, or that the woman with confusion and abnormal renal indices and normal vital signs actually has severe sepsis. It's recognizing that some patients who are responsive may well be in a coma by the next day.

Unfortunately, there's nothing in this book, or any other textbook, that will teach you this essential skill. And I have bad news for you—it won't be easy, it won't happen quickly, and it will take making lots of mistakes. Nevertheless, if you put in the effort, it will happen.

Your other goal for the rotation? Have fun. Seriously. You have trained for years to get to this point. You know your stuff. Now is the chance to see the extremes of pathophysiology and to experience all the acute care medicine that you have seen on TV and in the movies. It's also your chance to impress all your non-medical friends and family—after all, critical care is what they imagine every day in the hospital looks like.

- Try to learn something new every day. If this is your first ICU rotation, that shouldn't be difficult.
- Don't restrict the people you learn from to those in your discipline—if you are a medical intern, you can still learn a lot from a nurse or a respiratory therapist. Nurses can learn a lot from pharmacists.
- Don't panic. The unit staff know what they're doing, and this isn't their first rodeo.
- Read something every day.
  - Read while you're at the hospital. You spend enough time there. When you go home, focus on relaxing and recuperating.
  - Don't kid yourself and think that you'll read an entire chapter of a textbook every day. You won't, and even if you do, you won't absorb it. You can only learn 2-3 things at any given time.
  - There has never been a better time to get medical information. Blogs, Twitter, podcasts, Up To Date—these can be just as educational as a lecture or a textbook.
- Focus on the fundamentals. Read about the pathophysiology and treatment of respiratory failure, shock, hemorrhage, etc. Don't get too distracted by the esoteric stuff.

Rounding

Good rounding starts with good preparation. The key is to know your patient. That means more than just reviewing the labs and knowing the vital signs—it means knowing why he's in the ICU and how he's responding to the treatment you're providing.

Do your prerounding at the bedside. Most ICUs have plenty of computers available, either in each patient room or as a mobile workstation. Open the EMR and review all the labs and imaging. Examine the patient and look at all the infusions that are hanging and get the ventilator settings from the ventilator itself. Talk to the patient's nurse about anything that's happened over the last 24 hours and if there are any big plans for the day (going to the OR, imaging studies, etc.). Put in your orders and then move on to the next patient. If you make this your morning routine, you'll find that you're much more efficient and prepared than if you are constantly darting between the resident workroom and your patients' rooms.

When rounds start, you have three main objectives:
1. Convey the necessary information to the team about your patient and come up with the plan for the day.
2. Put in the necessary orders to make the plan happen.
3. Contribute to the education of the team (including yourself).

Convey the necessary information

This is what most people think of whey they talk about rounds. The intern relays any events over the last 24 hours, lists the vital signs and pertinent labs, describes her findings on physical exam, and then presents either a problem list or a breakdown by organ system. This is the format that has been followed for generations and is generally a good one as long as it's concise and focuses on the key findings.

Put in the necessary orders

Most ICUs nowadays have workstations on wheels that the team pushes around the unit during rounds. This is perfect for putting in orders. You should make sure that all the orders are placed before moving on to the next patient. This ensures it gets done and avoids confusion later ("I know we talked about Lasix. How much did we want? Or were we stopping Lasix?").

Contribute to the education of the team

Rounds are the time to discuss what you've been reading, or even to present an article to the team. Keep it short, though—there are a lot of patients to see, and a droning presentation will not be well-received. Hit the high points. This is also a good chance to ask questions about your patient to the fellow or attending. Ideally, the team should learn something new on every patient, every day.

The **prime question** that you should answer for every patient, every day, is this— *"Is he better, about the same, or worse today?"* While simple, the answer to the question will frame your entire assessment and plan. It relates to the overall trajectory of illness, not to any specific problem. After all, on any given day there will be some labs or imaging findings that are better than the day before, and some that are worse. Answering the prime question forces you to take a step back and to assess everything—the respiratory failure, shock, renal function, glycemic control, etc.

If the patient, on the whole, is getting better, then let him. Your plan is working (or at least not making him worse). Make the necessary adjustments but resist the urge to tinker too much with the plan of care.

If he's about the same, much of the above still applies. It's common in critical illness for the patient to plateau before he improves. That said, if there have been several days without any forward movement, it may be time to either change therapy or reexamine your diagnoses.

If the answer to the prime question is "getting worse," it means one of a few things. You may be missing something; there may be part of your plan that is causing toxicity or some other adverse side effect; or it may be the natural progression of the patient's disease that is resistant to treatment. In any event, if the patient is worse today, you need to reassess every part of your plan of care.

First, make sure you're not missing something. Reexamine your original assumptions about the diagnosis and investigate any new findings. Infection is a common complication in the ICU and can present in all sorts of ways that aren't typical. Pulmonary embolism, myocardial ischemia, and stroke all occur with regularity in the ICU and can occur without a textbook presentation.

Second, consider toxicity and side effects. Having a critical care PharmD can be invaluable here, as almost every medication we use in the ICU can have adverse effects. Nonpharmacologic therapies like mechanical ventilation, dialysis, and even simple things like nasogastric tubes and Foley catheters can all create problems.

Lastly, it may be that the patient's disease is progressing despite your best efforts. There's not much you can do here from a curative standpoint, although you should continue to provide adequate sedation, analgesia, and comfort measures.

The Great Debate—Problems vs. Systems

One of the first questions attendings get asked during the ICU rotation is, "How do you want us to present?" The answer depends a great deal on the unit culture and the attending's own preference, but it generally comes down to "by systems" or "by problems."

The problem list-based presentation follows the typical SOAP note[*] format. First, discuss any new developments over the last 24 hours, including the patient's input if he's able to communicate. Then, summarize the vital signs, pertinent findings on physical exam, and lab and imaging data. Finally, list the patient's diagnoses and problems, along with the current plan of care and any changes you want to make.

The problem list method is a good one because it emphasizes diagnosis and prompts you to commit to a plan. It's important to list the problems in some order of severity—acute respiratory failure, for example, should be listed ahead of hypokalemia.

The downside of the problem list is that you may miss the small but important things that need addressed. Be sure to cover nutrition, sedation and analgesia, DVT prophylaxis, mobility, and disposition.

---

[*] Subjective, Objective, Assessment, Plan

The systems-based presentation, on the other hand, seems to be unique to the ICU. Instead of providing a list of problems, you break things down by organ system. This ensures that all the areas are covered and is comprehensive in its approach. The typical list of systems is:

- Neurologic
- Cardiovascular
- Pulmonary/Respiratory
- Renal
- Gastrointestinal
- Endocrine
- Infectious Disease
- Hematologic
- Supportive Care (DVT prophylaxis, nutrition, mobility, etc.)

The downside of the systems method is that it's easy to miss the forest for the trees. Many an intern has gone through the entire presentation, describing each system, and then been stumped by the attending's question of, "So, what's wrong with her?" If you are using the system-based method, be sure to know the patient's underlying diagnoses as well.

The Importance of Diagnosis

Critical Care Medicine has a lot in common with Emergency Medicine. If a patient is crashing, the priorities are resuscitation and stabilization, not necessarily diagnosis. A critically ill patient needs respiratory, hemodynamic, and renal support regardless of the underlying illness. However, the importance of making an accurate and timely diagnosis should not be discounted. Without knowing the underlying cause of the patient's condition, necessary treatment may be delayed or not provided at all.

This has to be balanced with the patient's condition, of course. Leaving the ICU for any kind of diagnostic procedure can be risky. If a test is to be of benefit, it must provide *actionable information*—that is, the result obtained should be something that could change your treatment plan.

What This Book Is Not

Remember the part about reading something every day? Well, simply reading this book isn't enough. The information on these pages is presented in a way to help you on rounds and when you're working up your patient. This book isn't designed to be a review of critical care medicine. There are plenty of other textbooks, blog posts, podcasts, and other resources that will give you the foundational learning that you need. I've even put a list of the ones I find particularly helpful at the end of the book.

Instead, *The ICU Survival Book* is a compilation of the facts, formulas, tables, and troubleshooting that you'll need to be successful during your rotation. If you're having trouble with a particular issue, use the book to help work through it until you have the time to read up on the subject more thoroughly.

The following sections are grouped by systems, much like the system-based presentations that many ICUs use. Not every system is listed, and they aren't equally weighted—the sections on hemodynamics and respiratory care are more in-depth than the one covering nutrition. There's a list of things you should typically know on rounds, and then there's *What You Need To Survive.* These are the concepts, facts, and guidelines that get you through the rotation, provide a jumping-off point for further learning, and let you help some patients along the way.

If you're using the book appropriately, it should be full of your own notes and sketches by the end of your rotation. This is a tool, not a family heirloom. With any luck, you'll be able to come back to these pages as a review from time to time as you progress through your training.

Notes on Language and Attitude

This is something that I feel is important for clinicians, especially newcomers to the ICU. The language that we use when we're talking *about* patients will shape both the words and the attitudes we use when we're talking *to* patients and family members. It's very easy to get discouraged about what you're doing when you see so much disability, struggle, and even death on a daily basis. However, what we don't always see in the ICU are the patients who ultimately recover from critical illness or injury and go on to lead happy, fulfilling lives. The patient with the subdural hemorrhage who leaves the ICU with a tracheostomy and a feeding tube may very well walk back into your unit 6 months from now, under his own power, to thank the staff for saving his life. This doesn't mean everyone will pull through, and in fact many patients won't. But there will be enough patients who recover despite your negative predictions, and you will soon learn that it can be very difficult to accurately prognosticate early on. The older I get, the less confident I am in my ability to predict what will happen.

When you're speaking with family members, it's important to relay the seriousness of a patient's condition but be careful not to be overly pessimistic if it's still unclear what's likely to happen. Be honest with them and be honest with yourself. Sometimes the only correct answer is, "It's still too soon to know."

For every patient who recovers quickly, there will be another who needs weeks or months to get better. Recognize that there will be good days and bad days and don't get too discouraged with setbacks. Patients and families will pick up on your feelings, be them negative or positive, and that will have a significant impact on their own attitudes and decisions.

Be aware of the language you use. The ICU is a pretty dehumanizing place and it's important to preserve the dignity and humanity of the people we serve, even with the little things. For example, we procure organs—we don't "harvest" them. Harvesting is something farmers do with wheat. Organ donation is a gift, and we shouldn't cheapen it. Another thing—we don't "withdraw care" on patients. We withdraw ventilators, dialysis, and other life support measures, but we don't withdraw care.

If you use the term "withdraw care" with me, I know what you're talking about, and it doesn't hurt my feelings. But if that's what you say in rounds, at some point you're going to slip up and say it to a family. Their fear is that when they tell you to stop the ventilator/drips/etc., the patient will suffer and die alone with no one paying any attention to him. Using a term like "withdraw care" may cause them to reconsider a shift to comfort care. I can recall watching the face of a patient's son change when that phrase was said, and what had been a good therapeutic relationship suddenly became strained. He no longer trusted that we were going to do the right thing for his mother.

So, what to say? I think emphasizing what we really do is important. Something to this effect—

> *"You may hear the term 'withdraw care.' I want you to know that that's not what we do. Our priority is the relief of pain and suffering and we will make sure that happens even when the life support is removed. We will do our best to ensure that she receives all the care and dignity she deserves as a human being."*

As a critical care clinician, you are going to help some patients recover from one of the worst periods of their lives. You are going to help others to a peaceful, dignified death. Both are worthy endeavors. What you do here matters, even if it doesn't always feel like it.

I wrote the following ten years ago in the first edition of *The Ventilator Book*, and I believe them as much now as I did then—

Remember that your patient is a fellow human being with wants, needs, cares, and concerns that may be strikingly similar to your own. He deserves to be spoken to, even if he can't speak back. He deserves respect, even though he may not be able to return that respect. He deserves the basics of human kindness and touch. Remember that he has placed his life in your hands. Your job is not an easy one, and not one that most people can do. The recognition that you have positively affected the life of another person in a way that few can is the greatest reward of this great profession.

Hemodynamics

What To Know On Rounds

- Any vasoactive infusions (vasopressors, inotropes, antihypertensives)
- Blood pressure goals
- Dysrhythmias—tachycardias, bradycardias, blocks
- Assessment of oxygen delivery and consumption
- Right and left ventricular function
- Presence of myocardial ischemia or infarction

What You Need To Survive

The management of hemodynamics in the ICU is something that demands a great deal of time and attention. Most patients will require some sort of hemodynamic support during critical illness and it's important to understand the principles of blood pressure and organ system perfusion. This chapter covers:

- Blood pressure goals
- What to do when the blood pressure is too high
- Fluid and drug therapy for shock
- Cardiac filling pressures and cardiac output
- Types of shock
- A simplified, general approach to shock resuscitation
- Overview of dysrhythmias and treatment

Blood Pressure Goals

There is no one perfect blood pressure for ICU patients and trying to maintain the BP in an excessively tight range can be a fool's errand. It's better to adopt the Goldilocks approach—blood pressure shouldn't be too low, shouldn't be too high, but instead should be "about right." About right means that the vital organs are perfused, but the afterload isn't so high that it causes problems.

BP Too High

The systemic blood pressure is too high, and should be treated, when it's either causing or exacerbating end-organ damage. This is very different from the treatment of hypertension in otherwise stable outpatients, where the goal is prevention of long-term sequelae. In the ICU, the best approach to mildly elevated blood pressure is often to do nothing.

Types of End-Organ Damage Related to Hypertension
- Aortic dissection
- Cerebral edema
- Pulmonary edema
- Myocardial ischemia
- Glomerulonephritis with acute kidney injury
- Preeclampsia or eclampsia
- Intracerebral or subarachnoid hemorrhage

How Low To Go?

Condition	Hemodynamic Goals	Comments
Aortic dissection	SBP 100-120 HR 60-80	Goal is to prevent propagation of the dissection
Cerebral Edema Hypertensive Encephalopathy	Urgent reduction in MAP by 25%, then normalize BP over several days	Priority is cerebral perfusion
Pulmonary Edema	SBP < 140	Strategy is preload and afterload reduction, usually with diuretics and BP control
Myocardial Ischemia	SBP < 140 HR < 100	Endpoint is relief of chest pain

Acute Glomerulonephritis	Urgent reduction in MAP by 25%, then normalize BP over several days	Afterload reduction is the primary treatment
Preeclampsia Eclampsia	SBP < 160	Magnesium is the preferred agent for treatment
Intracerebral Hemorrhage	SBP 140-160	Goal is to prevent hematoma expansion
Subarachnoid hemorrhage	SBP 100-140	Goal is to prevent rerupture of aneurysm

Titratable Drugs That Make the Blood Pressure Go Down

Nicardipine	5-15 mg/hr infusion	calcium channel blocker; doesn't affect heart rate
Labetalol	10–20 mg IV push; 0.5-2 mg/min infusion	mixed α- and β-blocker; useful when you're trying to control both the heart rate and blood pressure
Esmolol	250-500 mcg/kg IV bolus; 50-200 mcg/kg/min infusion	primarily a β-1 selective blocker, with β-2 blockade at higher doses major advantage is a very short duration of action
Nitroglycerin	500-1000 mcg IV bolus, followed by 1-5 mcg/kg/min	vasodilator; improves coronary artery blood flow

BP Too Low

In general, the goal is to maintain a mean arterial pressure (MAP) of 65. This seems to be the necessary pressure, in most patients, to perfuse the organs. That doesn't mean that some patients (elderly, small body size, pregnant, cirrhotic, etc.) can't get by with a lower pressure, but if you choose a lower target you need to follow markers of perfusion closely. Other patients, particularly those with long-standing hypertension, may need a MAP *higher* than 65. Again, follow the markers of perfusion. If the patient is oliguric at a MAP of 65 but makes urine at 70, then increase the goal.

Markers of Good Perfusion

- Warm hands and feet
- Adequate urine output
- Appropriate mentation
- Brisk capillary refill (< 2 sec)
- Normal fetal heart rate
- Declining or normal lactate
- Declining or normal transaminases, renal indices, troponin

Fluid Resuscitation

Isotonic fluids are used as resuscitation fluids for hypotension and intravascular volume depletion. In general, these are best given as boluses (999 mL/hr on the IV pump, or via gravity with or without a pressure bag). The bolus is usually 500-1000 mL at a time, depending on the patient's size and the degree of hypotension. Once the patient has received 20-30 mL/kg of fluid, which is around 2-3 liters in most adult patients, you should evaluate his volume status in some way before giving more. This can be with bedside ultrasound, stroke volume variation (you will need an arterial line and a device like FloTrac or LidCO or PiCCO), or the humble physical exam.

With vasodilatory shock in particular, fluids can only get you so far. It's not a sign of weakness to start norepinephrine in a shocked patient! Even if the problem is primarily volume depletion, the norepinephrine will increase venous return and support the patient until he's fluid replete. The alternative, which is giving 8-10 liters or more before conceding that the patient is vasoplegic, can lead to problems down the line.

Remember that fluids, like drugs, all have beneficial effects and side effects. Gross fluid overload can lead to pulmonary, mesenteric, and peripheral edema, and may increase the risk of acute renal failure. Ideally, the fluid should be picked to match the patient's acid-base status, but recent studies have shown this doesn't have a significant effect on mortality so use what's available if your supply is limited.

Lactated Ringers (LR) is the fluid of choice most of the time in the ICU. It's nearly isotonic, has a pH of 6.5, and the lactate is metabolized to bicarbonate so it can actually help alkalinize the blood. There is a small amount of potassium (4 mEq/L), but *ample* research has shown that even large volumes of LR in the setting of renal failure will not lead to hyperkalemia. In fact, worsening acidemia is more likely to raise the serum potassium level.

Normal Saline (NS) is a 0.9% salt solution that is isotonic. It's also a good volume expander. The major drawback is that the high chloride content (154 mEq/L) can cause a significant hyperchloremic acidosis. This is usually well-tolerated, but a patient who already has a pH of 7.02 may not be able to handle the additional acidosis. If possible, reserve NS for patients with volume depletion and a contraction alkalosis (where the hyperchloremic fluid will be of benefit).

Sodium bicarbonate, when mixed as 150 mEq in one liter of sterile water, is also isotonic and can be used as a resuscitation fluid in patients with severe metabolic acidosis. Unfortunately, sodium bicarbonate is not shelf-stable and cannot be stored ahead of time in the ICU. It's worth giving if you have time to wait on the pharmacy to mix it up; use LR in the meantime.

Plasmalyte-A is a fluid that is designed to mirror the normal blood chemistry and has a pH of 7.40. Theoretically it should be the "ideal resuscitation fluid" but it's more expensive than LR or NS and is not as readily available. It is very useful if you're the neurotic type who can't stand seeing minor electrolyte abnormalities.

Drug Resuscitation[*]

Drug	Action	Dose	Comments
Norepinephrine	**α-agonist (peripheral vasoconstriction)** mild β1-agonist (chronotropy, inotropy)	0.05-2 mcg/kg/min 4–100 mcg/min[†]	generally the vasopressor of choice in most situations, and especially septic shock
Epinephrine	**β1-agonist (increases heart rate and contractility)** β2-agonist (bronchodilator, vasodilator) β3-agonist (increases blood glucose, lipolysis) α-agonist (increases peripheral vascular tone)	0.01-0.5 mcg/kg/min 1-40 mcg/min	main benefit in cardiogenic and septic shock is by increasing cardiac output drug of choice with anaphylactic shock at lower doses, effect on vascular resistance is less due to both α and β2 stimulation blood glucose and lactate levels are often high with epinephrine infusions

---

[*] For some reason, "resuscitation" has become a synonym for IV fluids— "the patient is under-resuscitated" typically means "I don't think you've given him enough fluid." That doesn't make sense—resuscitation means that the medical team has stabilized the patient's hemodynamic and respiratory status. Fluids may be the right answer, the wrong answer, or part of the answer. Resuscitation should refer to the whole picture.

[†] Typical doses are listed here in weight-based and non-weight-based doses, both of which are used in different institutions. There is no real "maximum" dose—titrate until you get the result you want, or a side effect you don't—but most ICUs will have dosing parameters established.

Phenylephrine	**α-agonist (peripheral vasoconstriction)**	0.5-3 mcg/kg/min 40-180 mcg/min	pure α-agonist with no effect on cardiac rate or contractility
			useful for vasoplegia, spinal shock
			do not use with aortic regurgitation—the increase in afterload will cause cardiac failure
Dopamine	**β1 and β2-agonist at lower doses** **α-agonist at higher doses** **D1-agonist (renal vasculature)***	5-20 mcg/kg/min	at less than 10 mcg/kg/min, the β activity is more pronounced. at a dose of 10-20 mcg/kg/min, the α activity is primary.
			dopamine can be useful as a pharmacologic pacer (increases hr) or when there is septic shock with significant systolic dysfunction
			tachyarrhythmias and extravasation risk are the major side effects

---

* Don't use dopamine for renal protection (AKA "renal dose dopamine"). Decades of research have shown that this doesn't help. Any improvement in renal function is due to the increase in cardiac output.

Dobutamine	**β1 and β2-agonist (increased chronotropy and inotropy; vasodilation)**	5-40 mcg/kg/min	primarily used as an inotrope can cause hypotension due to β2 activity
Milrinone	**PDE-3 inhibitor (inotropy and pulmonary vasodilation)**	0.125-0.75 mcg/kg/min	primarily used as an inotrope and with pulmonary hypertension less titratable with a longer duration of action, especially with renal failure
Vasopressin	**V1-agonist (vasoconstriction)** V2-agonist (renal, stimulates water retention) V3-agonist (CNS, stimulates ACTH)	0.01-0.04 units/min (typically 0.03 units/min) not titratable— think of it as a replacement hormone	adjunct to norepinephrine in septic shock stimulates nitric oxide release in coronary and pulmonary circulation, causing vasodilation can cause significant mesenteric and digital ischemia

| Hydrocortisone | **Glucocorticoid activity**

Mineralocorticoid activity (less pronounced) | 200-300 mg/day, either in divided doses or by continuous infusion | never-ending controversy in critical care medicine and no clear evidence for benefit

however, there is also little evidence for significant harm at the usual doses

it seems prudent to add hydrocortisone for adrenal support when a patient needs either high-dose or multiple vasopressors |

Cardiac Filling Pressures

Cardiac filling pressures tend to be low with hypovolemic and distributive shock and elevated with cardiogenic and obstructive pathology. The two filling pressures that are measured with a PA catheter are the central venous pressure (CVP) and the pulmonary artery occlusion pressure (PAOP). The CVP can also be measured with a central venous catheter placed in the superior vena cava (an IJ or subclavian line).

Since there are no valves between the vena cava and the right atrium, the CVP equals the right atrial pressure. The right atrial and ventricular pressures are the same at the end of diastole (when blood stops flowing from the atrium into the ventricle). Therefore, the **CVP = RVEDP**. If the CVP is elevated (> 8 mm Hg), this usually indicates right ventricular dysfunction.

The PAOP is measured with a PA catheter that is inserted into a segmental or subsegmental pulmonary artery. When the balloon on the catheter is inflated, blood flow in that artery stops and the tip of the catheter measures the pressure in the pulmonary capillary bed. The pressure in the pulmonary capillaries is the same as the pulmonary venous pressure, which is equivalent to the left atrial pressure. The left atrial pressure equals the left ventricular pressure at the end of diastole, so the **PAOP = LVEDP**. If the PAOP is elevated (> 16 mm Hg), this usually indicates left ventricular dysfunction.

The CVP and the PAOP are determined by blood volume and the function of the myocardium. They are **not** reflective of extracellular fluid status and should not be used in isolation to determine whether a patient needs fluids or diuresis. Rather, they should be used to evaluate the function of the right (CVP) and left (PAOP) ventricle at a given blood volume.

Cardiac filling pressures can be affected by other clinical conditions as well, so take all of these with a grain of salt. Some things that can elevate the CVP or PAOP and potentially mislead you:

- Positive pressure ventilation, especially with high PEEP or APRV
- Air trapping while on the vent (autoPEEP)
- Pericardial constriction
- Mitral regurgitation (the V wave seen when the balloon is inflated can make the PAOP seem higher than it is)
- Mitral stenosis (the PAOP reflects the LA pressure, but not the LVEDP)
- Tricuspid regurgitation (the V wave makes the CVP seem higher than it is; this can also affect the thermodilution-measured cardiac output)

Venous pressures can be evaluated, if not precisely measured, without a PA catheter or a central venous line. Since it's normal for venous pressure to be low, most abnormal findings will suggest elevated venous pressure (and concomitant ventricular dysfunction).

Surrogates For an Elevated CVP

- Distended neck veins
- Hepatojugular reflux
- Distended inferior vena cava on bedside ultrasound, without significant respiratory variation
  - o The diameter of the IVC should normally change by at least 50% with respiration in a patient not on the ventilator*
  - o The diameter of the IVC should normally change by 12-18% with respiration when the patient is on the ventilator
  - o IVC variation more than 18% during positive pressure ventilation suggests fluid responsiveness, but with a lot of ifs—*if* the tidal volume is 8-10 mL/kg, *if* the patient is making no respiratory efforts, and *if* there is no underlying RV dysfunction.

Surrogates For an Elevated PAOP

- Rales on pulmonary auscultation
- B-line predominance on bedside lung ultrasound (reflecting interstitial and alveolar edema)

Edema, ascites, and pleural effusions can be seen when there is acute RV or LV dysfunction but can also be seen when there is total body extracellular fluid overload without cardiogenic shock. That is, it's possible to have significant edema even with a normal CVP and PAOP.

---

* This reveals the folly of using IVC variation to guide fluid resuscitation in the non-ventilated patient. To give fluids until the IVC is "full" is another way of saying you'll give fluids until the patient has right atrial hypertension.

Cardiac Output

Cardiac output can be measured directly using a PA catheter or with a cardiac output monitor that uses the arterial waveform to measure stroke volume.[*] It can also be calculated using the Fick Equation. Cardiac output (CO) is better expressed as cardiac index (CI) by dividing the output by the patient's body surface area in m^2. Cardiac output can also be quantified as either "enough" or "not enough" with the physical exam and bedside ultrasound.

Surrogates For Inadequate CO ("Not Enough")
- Cold around the edges
- Weak peripheral pulses
- Narrow pulse pressure
- Oliguria
- Encephalopathy
- Poor LV and/or RV function on bedside ultrasound
- Rising lactate, transaminases, renal indices

Surrogates For Adequate CO ("Enough")
- Warm around the edges
- Bounding peripheral pulses
- Wide pulse pressure
- Good urine output
- Normal or hyperdynamic LV and/or RV function on bedside ultrasound
- Declining lactate, transaminases, renal indices

---

[*] Trade names for these monitors include FloTrac, LidCO, and PiCCO.

Thermodilution

A PA catheter has a thermometer that is located on the part of the catheter in the main pulmonary artery. If saline (either iced or room temperature) is injected into the right atrium or ventricle via a port on the catheter, it will cool the blood by a few degrees. As the heart pumps, this cool blood will eventually be circulated into the pulmonary arteries and the temperature of the blood measured at the thermometer will return to normal. The computer in the monitor measures the area under the curve[*] to calculate the cardiac output.

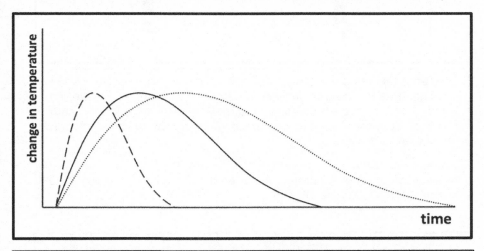

Solid line:	normal cardiac output
Dashed line:	high cardiac output (temperature returns to baseline faster)
Dotted line:	low cardiac output (temperature takes longer to return to baseline

---

[*] Called the Stewart-Hamilton equation, if you want a good trivia question.

Stroke Volume Variation

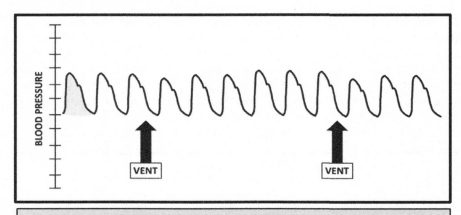

With an arterial blood pressure tracing, the stroke volume (SV) can be calculated as the area under the curve of the arterial pulse waveform (gray shading). If the patient is fluid-replete, or if the left ventricular function is depressed, there isn't much variation with positive pressure ventilation (arrows).

Cardiac output (CO) is the heart rate multiplied by the SV. This measurement is not accurate if the arterial waveform is irregular (atrial fibrillation, multiple PVCs).

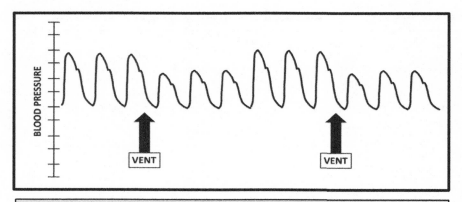

A stroke volume variation (SVV) with positive pressure ventilation > 15%) suggests that the patient may be fluid-responsive. The change in SV with ventilation reflects a drop in right ventricular preload, which then lowers the CO.

This measurement is less accurate when the tidal volume is less than 8-10 mL/kg or if the patient is breathing spontaneously.

Fick Equation

The Fick principle says that the patient will only consume as much oxygen as he needs, and the rest will not be absorbed from the alveoli. To measure this directly requires a nonrebreathing circuit with gas analyzers, which isn't practical in the ICU. Instead, we use the arteriovenous oxygen content difference (A-VO$_2$). The SaO$_2$ can be measured with an ABG. The SvO$_2$ is measured with a mixed venous blood gas drawn from the PA catheter.

$$\text{Oxygen Content (arterial blood)} = 1.34 \times Hgb \times SaO_2$$
$$\text{Oxygen Content (mixed venous blood)} = 1.34 \times Hgb \times SvO_2$$
$$\text{Oxygen Consumption (VO}_2\text{)} = CO \times [CaO_2 - CvO_2] \times 10^*$$

Expanded, this equation is:
$$VO_2 = CO \times [(1.34 \times Hgb \times SaO_2) - (1.34 \times Hgb \times SvO_2)] \times 10$$

Rearranged (and simpler):
$$VO_2 = CO \times 1.34 \times Hgb \times (SaO_2 - SvO_2) \times 10, \text{ or}$$
$$VO_2 = CO \times 13.4 \times Hgb \times (SaO_2 - SvO_2)$$

Indexing for body surface area:
$$VO_2I = CI \times 13.4 \times Hgb \times (SaO_2 - SvO_2)$$

Now, for the assumption—a normal VO$_2$I is about 125 mL O$_2$/min/m^2. That's in a healthy person at rest. This doesn't take into account things that can increase VO$_2$ like fever, sepsis, trauma, etc. But directly measuring the VO$_2$ is difficult, and the Fick Equation is useful as long as you keep in mind that the VO$_2$ is based on an assumption. Let's rearrange the equation one more time:

$$CI = VO_2I / [13.4 \times Hgb \times (SaO_2 - SvO_2)]$$

For a patient with a Hgb of 12 g/dL, SaO$_2$ of 99%, and SvO$_2$ of 74%:

$$CI = 125 / [13.4 \times 12 \times (0.99 - 0.74)]$$

$$CI = 3.1 \text{ L/min/m}^2$$

---

* Multiply by 10 to convert units—hemoglobin is measured in g/dL, while cardiac output is measured in L/min

Systemic Vascular Resistance

It's misleading to talk about measuring the systemic vascular resistance (SVR), since it can't be measured directly. It's also misleading to correlate SVR with arterial afterload and to initiate treatment based on this calculation. SVR is simply the relationship between blood flow (cardiac output), mean arterial pressure, and the central venous pressure and is a useful shorthand to refer to the degree of peripheral vasoconstriction present.

SVR is calculated following Ohm's Law, which states that the resistance equals the voltage divided by current. Substituting the pressure drop (MAP – CVP) for voltage, and cardiac output (CO) for current, we get

$$SVR = (MAP - CVP) / CO$$

Of these parameters, the cardiac output is the biggest driver. The SVR is typically high when the cardiac output is low, and vice versa. A normal SVR is 10-15 Wood units.[*] If the cardiac index is used instead of the cardiac output (which is preferred), the normal SVRI is 20-30 Wood units.

Clinically, we can use this concept to evaluate the adequacy of perfusion. First, if the SVR is elevated, then there is generally peripheral vasoconstriction. Cold fingers and toes, poor capillary refill, and mottling—"cold around the edges"—are all signs of a high SVR. A low SVR is associated with being "warm around the edges"—brisk capillary refill, warm toes, good skin perfusion.

Second, and this is very important—the SVR depends primarily on the cardiac output. If the SVR is high (cold around the edges), it indicates inadequate cardiac output. If the patient is warm around the edges, indicating a normal or low SVR, the cardiac output is usually normal or elevated. Treatment of a high SVR should not focus on treating vasoconstriction with vasodilators, but instead should focus on increasing the cardiac output.

---

[*] Calculating Wood units (named after Dr. Paul Wood, the "foremost British cardiologist of the 20th century") is pretty easy and intuitive. I don't see why you need to multiply by 79.9 to get dyne-sec-cm^{-5}, but if that's how your unit rolls, do the math.

Pulmonary Vascular Resistance

Calculating PVR is just like calculating SVR, except that you use the pressure drop over the pulmonary vasculature.

$$PVR = (mean\ PA\ pressure - PAOP)\ /\ CO.$$

$$PVRI = (mPAP - PAOP)\ /\ CI.$$

A normal PVR is 2-3 Wood units; a normal PVRI is 4-6 Wood units.

The main utility of the PVR is figuring out if pulmonary hypertension is due to things that increase pulmonary arterial pressures (like primary pulmonary hypertension, connective tissue disease, thromboembolic disease, etc.) or secondary to either elevated left ventricular pressure (e.g., CHF) or high cardiac output.

Types of Shock

There are five different mechanisms of shock, which all lead to the final common pathway of inadequate tissue oxygenation and impaired metabolic function. There can be considerable overlap of mechanisms, due to either the primary disease process or the patient's underlying health problems.

Mechanisms of Shock

- Cardiogenic (left ventricular, right ventricular, or biventricular)
- Hypovolemic (hemorrhagic or non-hemorrhagic)
- Distributive (vasoplegia due to sepsis, anaphylaxis, adrenal insufficiency, or loss of spinal function)
- Obstructive (cardiac tamponade, tension pneumothorax, high intrathoracic or intraabdominal pressure, massive pulmonary embolism)
- Cytopathic (inability of the mitochondria to use the delivered oxygen)

The combination of physical exam and bedside ultrasound can often determine the primary mechanism of shock. Most critical care textbooks will have a table of the different shock states along with the measured or calculated data from a pulmonary artery (PA) catheter. While this is useful for board exams, it's not too helpful in the 21st century ICU where PA catheters are few and far between.

Fortunately, it's easy to substitute those parameters for some easily obtainable physical exam and bedside ultrasound findings.

Cardiogenic Shock

PA Catheter Parameters	Physical Exam Findings	Bedside Ultrasound
CVP elevated (> 8 mm Hg)	neck veins distended	dilated IVC with low respiratory variation
PAOP elevated (> 16 mm Hg)	rales on lung exam	B-line predominance in lungs
SVRI elevated (> 30 Wood units)	cold around the edges	
CI low (< 2.2 L/min/m^2)	poor organ system perfusion	sluggish or poor LV and/or RV function adequate ventricular volume

Hypovolemic Shock

PA Catheter Parameters	Physical Exam Findings	Bedside Ultrasound
CVP low (< 5 mm Hg)	neck veins flat	small-diameter IVC with significant respiratory variation
PAOP low (< 10 mm Hg)	clear lung exam	A-line predominance in lungs
SVRI elevated (> 30 Wood units)	cold around the edges	
CI low (< 2.2 L/min/m^2)	poor organ system perfusion	hyperdynamic LV and RV function underfilled ventricles

Distributive Shock

PA Catheter Parameters	Physical Exam Findings	Bedside Ultrasound
CVP low (< 5 mm Hg)	neck veins flat	small-diameter IVC with significant respiratory variation
PAOP low (< 10 mm Hg)	clear lung exam	A-line predominance in lungs
SVRI low (< 20 Wood units)	warm around the edges	
CI normal or high (> 2.2 L/min/m²)	poor organ system perfusion	hyperdynamic LV function

Obstructive Shock

PA Catheter Parameters	Physical Exam Findings	Bedside Ultrasound
CVP elevated (> 8 mm Hg)	neck veins distended	dilated IVC with low respiratory variation
PAOP can be low or high Cardiac tamponade—PA diastolic and PAOP about the same as the CVP (equalization of diastolic pressures: RVEDP = PAD = LVEDP	clear lung exam asymmetric breath sounds with tension pneumothorax	A-line predominance in lungs absence of pleural sliding with tension pneumothorax pericardial effusion with diastolic collapse in cardiac tamponade
SVRI elevated (> 30 Wood units)	cold around the edges	

CI low (< 2.2 L/min/m^2)	poor organ system perfusion	hyperdynamic LV function with dilated, hypokinetic RV (pulmonary embolism)
	muffled heart tones with cardiac tamponade	pericardial effusion with atrial or ventricular collapse during diastole (cardiac tamponade)
	abdominal distension with compartment syndrome	underfilled ventricles, hyperdynamic function (abdominal compartment syndrome, tension pneumothorax)

Cytopathic Shock

Cytopathic shock is often a final common pathway with refractory distributive shock; it can also be seen with certain poisonings that uncouple oxidative phosphorylation like cyanide and salicylates. Features include refractory hypotension; coma; pronounced lactic acidosis; and a very high SvO$_2$ (indicating minimal tissue oxygen extraction and utilization).

Simplified Approach to Shock

Obviously, the right answer to "how should I resuscitate this patient in shock" is a very individual one that depends on the underlying cause, cardiac function, comorbidities, etc. However, it's helpful to have an approach that works most of the time while you're trying to sort things out.

Keep in mind that a patient may initially respond and then decline. Flow may seem adequate, and then it isn't. Conditions that weren't present beforehand now may be. Frequent monitoring and reassessment are key parts of any resuscitation.

Additionally, the flowchart listed here just addresses the hemodynamic part of things. Equally important is respiratory support. A deteriorating, shocky patient will often need intubation as a part of the resuscitation and you shouldn't wait for the ABG to look bad or the SpO$_2$ to drop before you intervene.

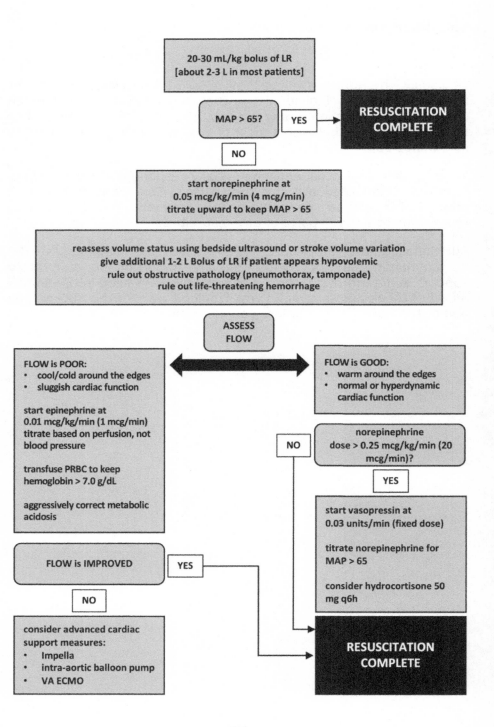

Dysrhythmias

Dysrhythmias can be grouped into two major categories—too fast and too slow. Both categories can be treated with drugs and electricity. The treatment, obviously, depends on how unstable the patient is. This section is not intended to be exhaustive—you're encouraged to review one of the many great books on ECG interpretation to learn the basics, and then interpret a lot of ECGs to get good at it.

Dysrhythmias are common in the ICU and tend to cause problems once the heart rate (HR) exceeds 150-160 beats per minute (bpm) or is less than 50 bpm. In general, it's a good idea to check the following whenever a patient develops a new dysrhythmia:

- 12-lead ECG
- Pulse oximeter—make sure airway and breathing are OK!
- Serum electrolytes—in particular, potassium, calcium, and magnesium levels
- The medication list

It's helpful to subdivide the different dysrhythmias based on rate, regularity, and the width of the QRS complex. This quickly narrows the differential and makes diagnosis and treatment easier.

Differential Diagnosis When the Rate Is Too Fast (HR > 100, and typically a lot faster than that)

Regular rhythm, Narrow QRS (< 120 msec)

- Sinus tachycardia
    - o The most common, and the treatment should focus on the underlying cause
- Atrial tachycardia
    - o Originates from an ectopic atrial pacemaker and is typically faster than sinus tachycardia (usually > 160 bpm).
    - o A P wave is present but has a different morphology than the usual sinus rhythm P wave.
    - o Treatment is with beta-blockers or calcium channel blockers.
- Atrial flutter
    - o Has characteristic saw-toothed flutter waves, but these can be difficult to see when the heart rate is high.

35

- o Consider atrial flutter when the rate is sticking right around 150—the flutter waves are typically 300/min, with 2:1 conduction slowing at the AV node.
- o Treatment is with beta-blockers or calcium channel blockers. Goal HR is < 120 bpm.
- o Atrial flutter will often break to sinus rhythm or progress to atrial fibrillation.
- o Synchronized cardioversion with 50-100 J can be used for significantly unstable patients, but this usually isn't successful.
- Supraventricular tachycardia (SVT)
  - o This can be due to an accessory pathway in the AV node or in the AV valvular rings.
  - o There is no P wave before the QRS complex because it's like a short-circuit in the AV node. The rate is typically high—170-190 bpm.
  - o Adenosine (6-12 mg IVP) is a good way to treat—it blocks the reentrant conduction pathway and allows the heart to reset into sinus rhythm.
  - o Beta-blockers and calcium channel blockers can be used for rate control—if you can keep the HR < 150, the short circuit will often terminate, and sinus rhythm will take over.
  - o Synchronized cardioversion with 50-100 J for unstable patients.
- Junctional Tachycardia
  - o Fairly uncommon and often associated with medications like digoxin or theophylline
  - o P waves may be inverted or behind the QRS complex due to retrograde conduction.
  - o Treatment is with amiodarone.

Irregular rhythm, Narrow QRS

- Atrial fibrillation
  - o The most common cause of an irregular rhythm in the ICU.
  - o No P waves are evident, just a fibrillating baseline between beats
  - o Treatment is with amiodarone, beta-blockers, or calcium channel blockers. Goal HR is < 120 bpm.
  - o Synchronized cardioversion with 100-200 J for unstable patients; try to load with amiodarone first

(150 mg IV) to make it more likely to convert the rhythm.
- Atrial flutter with variable conduction
    - This is a "regularly irregular" rhythm.
    - Flutter waves are seen between the QRS complexes.
    - Treatment is the same as for regular atrial flutter.
- Multifocal atrial tachycardia
    - At least three different-appearing P waves will be seen in Lead II
    - Usually associated with COPD exacerbations
    - Treatment is rate control with calcium channel blockers, with a goal HR < 120 bpm, and treatment of the COPD exacerbation

Regular rhythm, Wide QRS (> 120 msec)
- Ventricular Tachycardia
    - By far, the most common and most potentially lethal wide-complex tachycardia
    - Treatment is with amiodarone or lidocaine for stable patients, but be ready to cardiovert at any time.
    - Synchronized cardioversion with 100-200 J for unstable patients
- SVT with aberrant conduction
    - SVT in the setting of known conduction delay
    - There are criteria for it, but they're difficult to remember and even cardiologists don't always agree
    - Keep it simple—the treatments for ventricular tachycardia will also work for SVT with aberrancy. If you treat VT like SVT, however, bad things could happen. Approach all regular wide-complex tachycardia like it's VT.

Irregular rhythm, Wide QRS
- Accessory pathway conduction—this will look like atrial fibrillation but with a very high rate (usually > 200 bpm)
    - Immediate cardioversion, 100-200 J, is often the best and safest treatment
    - Procainamide or amiodarone can also be used if the patient is stable

37

- Polymorphic Ventricular Tachycardia (a.k.a. Torsades de Pointes)
  - Characterized by the twisting appearance of the QRS complex
  - Treatment is with magnesium sulfate
  - Amiodarone and procainamide may exacerbate the long QT interval and not be helpful
  - Replace potassium, aiming for a K > 4.5 mEq/L
  - Defibrillation (**not** cardioversion) 200 J for unstable patients—the defibrillator will not sync to the variable QRS complexes

Common Causes of Bradycardia (HR < 50)
- Hypoxemia (very common)
- Medications (beta blockers, calcium channel blockers, digitalis, propofol, cholinergic drugs)
- Hyperkalemia
- Hypermagnesemia
- Hypocalcemia
- Hypothermia
- Metabolic acidosis
- Increased intracranial pressure (Cushing's reflex)
- Acute myocardial infarction (anterior wall and inferior wall MI can both affect the AV node)
- Infective endocarditis with a valvular abscess
- Sick sinus syndrome
- Hypothyroidism

Treatment consists of stabilizing cardiac function while addressing the underlying cause. Stabilizing cardiac function can be done using drugs, electricity, or both. Get a 12-lead ECG to look for any conduction blocks.

Medications For Bradycardia
- Atropine
  - Blocks vagus nerve conduction
  - Ineffective in complete heart block
  - Contraindicated s/p heart transplant—may cause asystole

- Epinephrine
  - Preferred medical therapy
  - Can be given as a push dose of 10-20 mcg IV during resuscitation
  - Infusion of 2-10 mcg/min is very effective
- Dopamine
  - Readily available in premixed bags
  - 5-10 mcg/kg/min is the typical dose
- Calcium
  - Helpful for medication-induced and electrolyte-induced bradycardia
  - 1 gram calcium chloride IV
  - 3 grams calcium gluconate IV

Emergency Transcutaneous Pacing[*]

- Apply pads and set to "Demand" mode unless the patient is periarrest or in cardiac arrest ("Fixed" mode is necessary in these situations)
- Administer sedation and analgesia, if appropriate
- Cardiac arrest, or comatose patient:
  - Set the rate to 80 bpm
  - Start pacing at the highest output (200 mA), and reduce the output after capture has been achieved.
  - The pacing threshold is the point where capture is lost—increase the output to 5-10 mA over the threshold
- Conscious patient:
  - Start pacing at 10 mA and increase by 5-10 mA at a time until there is capture
  - The pacing threshold is the point where capture is lost—increase the output to 5-10 mA over the threshold
- Successful capture is defined as a QRS complex and T wave following the pacer spike, **and** a peripheral pulse

---

[*] This presumes that you either know how to do this procedure or are in the company of someone who does.

Respiratory Failure

What To Know On Rounds

- Is the patient on a ventilator?
- Why is he on the ventilator?
- What are the current settings, and have there been any major adjustments in the last 24 hours?
- Is today a ventilator day? If so, what settings need to be adjusted? Is the patient being ventilated safely?
- If it's a get off the ventilator day, what needs to happen for him to be extubated?
- Are there any pulmonary issues that need treatment?

What You Need To Survive

Respiratory failure is the most common reason for admission to the ICU. Here, we'll focus on mechanical ventilation and troubleshooting. This section covers:

- What a ventilator can and cannot do to treat respiratory failure
- A glossary of terms used with mechanical ventilation
- An overview of common modes of ventilation
- Initial vent settings based on pathophysiology
- Noninvasive positive pressure ventilation
- Tidal volume and PEEP tables
- Troubleshooting different situations
- A flowchart for airway management

THREE THINGS A VENTILATOR CAN DO

1. Provide an FiO_2 as high as 100%
   - Even though the gas coming out of the wall is 100% oxygen, noninvasive respiratory support modes like high-flow nasal cannula and BiPAP still have leaks that allow some atmospheric air to be entrained.
   - With a cuffed endotracheal tube, the ventilator can reliably provide oxygen, up to 100%.

2. Use positive pressure to reduce intrapulmonary shunt
   - Pulmonary shunt refers to areas of lung that are perfused, but not ventilated. Think of a patient with a mucus plug and complete atelectasis of an entire lung—blood is still flowing through, but there's no gas exchange. Hypoxemia will ensue.
   - Most disease processes that cause respiratory failure are associated with shunt—pulmonary edema, ARDS, pneumonia, aspiration pneumonitis, etc. Positive pressure ventilation can open up and stabilize diseased alveoli, reduce shunt, and improve oxygenation.

3. Take over the work of breathing
   - This is intuitive with hypercapnic respiratory failure—the respiratory muscles are too weak to ventilate CO_2 and mechanical ventilation is necessary.
   - This is less intuitive, but no less true, when the work of breathing is too much for the patient to maintain. Septic shock, multisystem trauma, and acute heart failure may not cause hypercapnia but impose an excessive work of breathing. Recognition of impending respiratory failure and early intubation is always preferable to waiting for the patient to crash.

ONE THING A VENTILATOR CANNOT DO

Make a patient get better faster
- The ventilator is a means of support and will help keep the patient alive while the underlying cause of respiratory failure is being treated.
- The ventilator settings themselves cannot make the patient get better—it's not a combination lock.

THREE THINGS TO CONSIDER FOR VENTILATED PATIENTS

1. Don't hurt the patient with injurious ventilator settings
    *   While the ventilator may not make the patient get better any faster, it sure can hurt him if the pressures or tidal volumes are too high. Here are some general safety limits for mechanical ventilation[*]:
        o   Use a physiologic tidal volume, which is usually 4-8 mL/kg predicted body weight.[†] In ARDS, keep the tidal volume in the 4-6 mL/kg range.
        o   Keep the end-inspiratory alveolar pressure, or plateau pressure, at 30 or less.
        o   Keep the driving pressure (plateau pressure – end expiratory pressure, or P_{PLAT} – PEEP) in the 10-15 range if possible. Try very hard to not let it exceed 18-20.
        o   Routinely check for auto-PEEP and adjust the ventilator to minimize or eliminate it.
    *   Remember that your goal is not a perfect ABG. While the ventilator should be used to provide adequate gas exchange, the key word is "adequate."
        o   While a normal PaO_2 is 100, a PaO_2 of 65 is acceptable. Most of the time, a PaO_2 of 55-90 (which correlated with an SpO_2 of 88-96%) is sufficient.
        o   Mild respiratory acidosis is generally well-tolerated. A pH of 7.25 and a $PaCO_2$ of 52 is preferred if the alternative is using too high of a tidal volume in order to normalize these.
        o   "Perfect is the enemy of good" applies to most of what we do in the ICU.

2. Don't let the patient wear himself out
    *   Provide enough ventilator support to make the patient comfortable.

----

[*] This obviously does not apply to every situation, but these limits are generally useful.

[†] The predicted body weight (PBW) is based on the patient's height and gender. **You must know this on all ventilated patients.** Do not use the actual body weight to set the tidal volume!

- During acute cardiopulmonary failure, shock, etc. it is usually necessary to take over the work of breathing almost entirely.

3. Take him off the ventilator when he's ready
    - Every day is either a "vent day" or a "get off the vent day."
    - If it's a "vent day," adjust the settings to provide adequate gas exchange and make sure that you're within the safety limits. Be sure that the patient is comfortable.
    - If it's a "get off the vent day," do a spontaneous breathing trial. If the patient passes, extubate him.
    - In order for it to be a "get off the vent day," the following will usually* apply:
        o The underlying reason for respiratory failure should be getting better
        o The FiO_2 is 0.5 or lower
        o The PEEP is 8 or lower
        o There is no significant auto-PEEP
        o The patient is not requiring a high degree of hemodynamic support—high-dose or multiple vasopressors, mechanical cardiac support, etc.
        o The patient can respond and follow directions.
        o Protective airway reflexes (cough) are present, and secretions aren't excessive
    - If you never reintubate a patient, you're waiting too long and some of your patients are spending more time on the vent than they have to. If you reintubate 40-50% of the people you extubate, you're not being cautious enough. A 10-20% reintubation rate is probably about right.

---

* "Usually" does not mean "always." You have to consider the patient's baseline health status and other factors.

MECHANICAL VENTILATION PARAMETERS AND TERMS

Rate: the number of breaths that a patient will receive a minute. This can either be the set rate on the ventilator, or the total rate (ventilator breaths plus patient-triggered breaths).

Tidal Volume (VT): the amount of gas that a patient receives during a breath. A typical tidal volume is 5-8 mL/kg of the predicted body weight (PBW). In ARDS, the tidal volume is usually kept between 4-6 mL/kg PBW. In less severe cases of respiratory failure, the tidal volume is set between 6-8 mL/kg PBW. Patients with asthma and COPD often have above-average air hunger and may need a tidal volume as high as 8-10 mL/kg PBW.

Minute Ventilation: the rate multiplied by the tidal volume. The minute ventilation determines how much CO_2 is ventilated. The higher the minute ventilation, the lower the $PaCO_2$.

FiO_2: the fraction of inspired oxygen, referred to either as a percentage (e.g., 40%) or as a number (e.g., 0.4). Contrary to popular belief, the ventilator will go as low as room air—FiO_2 0.21. Oxygen is like any other drug in the ICU—use as much as the patient needs, but not any more than that.

PaO_2/FiO_2 Ratio (or P/F ratio, for short): divide the PaO_2 (in mm Hg) by the FiO_2 (as a number). This indexes the PaO_2 to the amount of inspired oxygen. A PaO_2 of 100 while breathing room air has a PaO_2/FiO_2 ratio of 100/0.21, or 476. A PaO_2 of 60 on an FiO_2 of 100% has a PaO_2/FiO_2 ratio of 60/1.0, or 60.

PEEP: PEEP stands for "positive end-expiratory pressure." It's the pressure that the ventilator continues to apply to the lungs once the breath is over. PEEP can be used to reduce pulmonary shunting (and improve oxygenation) by opening up collapsed or flooded alveoli. PEEP is generally set between 5 and 20 cm H_2O, depending on how severe the hypoxemia is.

CPAP: CPAP stands for "continuous positive airway pressure." For all intents and purposes, it's the same thing as PEEP. We generally use the term PEEP when the ventilator is doing the breathing and CPAP when the patient is doing the breathing.

Pressure Support (PS): the inspiratory pressure that the ventilator gives the patient when he triggers a breath, either in SIMV or PSV mode. Think of PS as a boost. Some patients have strong lungs and won't need much of a boost at all to breathe comfortably (maybe 0-5 cm PS); others aren't as strong and need more of a boost to get a decent tidal volume (15-20 cm PS). The PS can be adjusted up and down based on the patient's efforts in order to keep the spontaneous rate and tidal volume in a comfortable range.

Spontaneous Breathing Trial (SBT): when you think the patient is potentially ready for extubation, an SBT is performed to see how he breathes with little or no support. An SBT is often done in one of two ways:

- A PS/CPAP trial using a PS of 5-8 cm and a CPAP of 0-8 cm. This is enough support to overcome the resistance of the tubing, but it still requires the patient to do the majority of the work of breathing. The advantage is that the clinician can see the rate and tidal volume on the ventilator. The disadvantage is that the ventilator still provides some degree of support, which may mask underlying respiratory weakness.

- A T-piece (or T-tube) trial involves disconnecting the ventilator entirely and connecting the endotracheal tube to blow-by oxygen using a T-shaped adapter. The advantage of the T-piece trial is that it allows you to see how the patient does without any vent support (which can be especially helpful with hypercapnic respiratory failure). The disadvantage is that you can't readily measure the respiratory rate and tidal volume.

Plateau Pressure (P_{PLAT}): the pressure measured at the end of an inspiratory hold maneuver. The P_{PLAT} reflects the alveolar pressure at end-inspiration. In most cases, try to keep the P_{PLAT} less than 30 to prevent ventilator-induced lung injury.

Driving Pressure (ΔP): the pressure required to inflate the alveoli, starting from the end-expiratory pressure. This can be calculated as: P_{PLAT} − PEEP. In ARDS, a driving pressure > 15 is associated with higher mortality. Try to keep the driving pressure in the 10-15 range.

Peak Inspiratory Pressure (PIP):   the pressure needed to deliver the tidal volume during the time set for inspiration. The PIP represents both the pressure needed to inflate the alveoli and the pressure needed to overcome the resistance of the tubing and the patient's airways.

Auto-PEEP: when the alveoli don't empty completely during expiration, pressure can build up. When this pressure is higher than the set PEEP on the vent, it's known as breath-stacking, dynamic hyperinflation, or auto-PEEP. This can be measured during an expiratory hold maneuver. It's most commonly seen in patients with obstructive airway disease like asthma and COPD. Auto-PEEP can lead to increased dead space, which makes the $PaCO_2$ rise.

Modes Of Ventilation

Mode	Key Features	When Is It Useful?
Assist-Control (Volume) Also Known As: • CMV • PRVC • VC+ • VCV	You set a rate and a tidal volume, which the patient is guaranteed to receive. If he wants to breathe more than the set rate, he gets the full tidal volume every time.	This is the mode of choice most of the time in the ED or ICU because it takes over the work of breathing almost entirely. Many clinicians prefer to set the tidal volume (which makes the inspiratory pressure variable).
Assist-Control (Pressure) (PCV)	You set a rate, an inspiratory pressure, and an inspiratory time. If the patient wants to breathe over the set rate, he can—he'll get the inspiratory pressure for the set inspiratory time.	This is like volume assist-control, except that the pressure is set and so the tidal volume is variable. This mode is useful in some patients with ARDS where you're concerned about keeping the driving pressure controlled.
Synchronized Intermittent Mandatory Ventilation (SIMV, or SIMV/PS)	The rate and tidal volume (or inspiratory pressure, if selected) is guaranteed. If the patient wants to breathe over the set rate, he has to pull whatever volume he can. Spontaneous breaths can be augmented with Pressure Support.	SIMV is useful when the patient wants to breathe on his own and has some cardiopulmonary reserve. The Pressure Support can be adjusted to keep the patient-generated rate and tidal volume in a comfortable range. As the patient takes on more of the workload, the machine rate can be lowered.

48

Pressure Support Ventilation (PSV, or PS/CPAP)	There is no set rate with PSV, just a Pressure Support. The patient has to trigger all of his own breaths. The Pressure Support augments his inspiratory efforts.	PSV requires the patient to be able to initiate all of his own breaths, so it's typically used during recovery. It can also be used when the intrinsic drive to breathe is very high— severe metabolic acidosis, for example.
Airway Pressure Release Ventilation Also Known As: • APRV • Bi-Vent • Bi-Level	APRV uses a prolonged time at a high pressure to open up flooded alveoli, followed by a very brief drop in pressure that allows CO_2 to be ventilated but short enough to keep alveoli from collapsing.	APRV is designed for ARDS and other diffuse, bilateral, restrictive lung disease. It can let you increase the mean airway pressure and improve oxygenation without using excessively high distending pressures and may help prevent ventilator-induced lung injury in severe ARDS.

Initial Ventilator Settings Based on Pathophysiology[*]

Restrictive Lung Disease

Examples: ARDS, aspiration pneumonitis, pneumonia, pulmonary fibrosis, pulmonary edema, alveolar hemorrhage, chest trauma

Restrictive lung diseases are associated with a reduction in respiratory system compliance. The lungs want to collapse. In other words, it's hard to get air in and easy to get air out. The ventilation strategy is to recruit vulnerable alveoli, prevent cyclical alveolar closure, provide adequate oxygenation, and to minimize volutrauma from overdistension.

---

[*] Taken from *The Ventilator Book*, 3rd Edition.

The initial mode should be one that takes over the work of breathing for the patient. Assist-control, using either volume-controlled or pressure-controlled ventilation, is the mode of choice.

For volume-controlled ventilation:
1. Tidal volume of 6 mL/kg PBW
2. Rate of 14-18 breaths per minute, with a decelerating flow pattern
3. FiO_2 100% at first; reduce to 60% if $SpO_2 \geq 88\%$
4. PEEP of 5-10 cm H_2O, depending on the degree of hypoxemia. Remember, the more opacification in the lungs on the chest X-ray, the more PEEP will be needed to reduce intrapulmonary shunting.
5. If hypoxemia persists, increase the PEEP until the SpO_2 is 88% or better. Don't exceed 20.
6. After adjusting the PEEP, check the plateau pressure. If the P_{PLAT} is more than 30 cm H_2O, decrease the tidal volume until the P_{PLAT} is less than 30. Don't go below 4 mL/kg PBW.

For pressure-controlled ventilation:
1. PEEP of 5-10 cm H_2O, depending on the degree of hypoxemia
2. FiO_2 100%; reduce to 60% if $SpO_2 \geq 88\%$
3. Inspiratory pressure of 15-20 cm H_2O
4. Rate of 14-18 breaths per minute
5. Inspiratory time adjusted to keep the I:E ratio 1:1.5 or higher. The I-time is usually 1.0-1.5 seconds. A rate of 20 and an I-time of 1.0 seconds has an I:E ratio of 1:2 (one second inspiration, two seconds expiration). A rate of 15 with an I-time of 1.5 seconds has an I:E ratio of 1:1.7 (1.5 seconds inspiration, 2.5 seconds expiration). This is displayed on the ventilator screen.
6. If hypoxemia persists, increase the PEEP until the SpO_2 is 88% or better. Don't exceed 20 cm H_2O.
7. Look at the exhaled tidal volume. If it exceeds 6 mL/kg, lower the inspiratory pressure until the tidal volume is in the 4-6 mL/kg range.

After initiating ventilation, check an arterial blood gas. 15-20 minutes is enough time for gas exchange to equilibrate.

Make changes in the respiratory rate to change the $PaCO_2$ (a higher rate lowers the $PaCO_2$, and vice versa). Leave the tidal volume in the 4-6 mL/kg range, keeping the P_{PLAT} at 30 cm H_2O or less. Remember that lung protection is more important than normal ventilation—a pH of 7.15 or better is acceptable and it's not worth injuring the lungs with overdistension (in the form of high tidal volumes) to get a normal pH or $PaCO_2$.

Lower the FiO_2, keeping the PaO_2 between 55- and 90-mm Hg and the SpO_2 between 88% and 94%. There's nothing to gain from keeping the PaO_2 above this range, with few exceptions. Patients with traumatic brain injury sometimes require a higher PaO_2, usually in conjunction with brain tissue oxygen monitoring. Victims of carbon monoxide poisoning also benefit from breathing 100% oxygen.

Obstructive Airways Disease

Examples: COPD, Asthma

Obstructive lung disease is associated with an increase in respiratory system compliance and an obstruction to expiratory airflow. <u>It's easy to get air in, but hard to get it out.</u>

The ventilation strategy is to rest the respiratory muscles, provide adequate oxygenation, and reduce hyperinflation.

Assist-control ventilation is usually the mode of choice, and volume-control is preferable to pressure-control. SIMV with PS can also be used, however, so long as the rate and PS are set high enough to prevent tachypnea and fatigue. High airway resistance and high peak inspiratory pressures characterize exacerbations of COPD and asthma, even though the P_{PLAT} may be significantly lower. Using pressure-control in this situation leads to very low tidal volumes. Volume-control guarantees that the desired tidal volume will be delivered.

1. Tidal volume of 8 mL/kg PBW. Lower tidal volumes can lead to air trapping and worsening hyperinflation.
2. Rate of 10-14 breaths per minute
3. Inspiratory time adjusted to keep an I:E ratio of 1:3 or higher. In obstructive airways disease, air gets in easily but has a hard time getting out due to narrow, inflamed bronchioles and bronchi. Give the air some time to escape.
4. With asthma, applied PEEP will worsen hyperinflation. With COPD, PEEP can be used to splint open airways that are prone to collapse. This is because COPD is characterized by dynamic airway obstruction, while the obstruction is fixed in an asthma exacerbation. A good starting point for both is a PEEP of 0, or ZEEP—zero applied end-expiratory pressure.
5. FiO_2 of 100% to start; lower this to 60% if the SpO_2 remains 88% or better.

Sometimes, patients with COPD or asthma will remain tachypneic despite adequate sedation. In assist-control, every patient-triggered breath delivers a full tidal volume, and this can lead to air trapping or severe respiratory alkalosis. If this is the case, switching the mode to SIMV may help.

Severe Metabolic Acidosis

Examples: Salicylate poisoning, septic shock, toxic exposures, acute renal failure, diabetic ketoacidosis

The normal response of the respiratory system in the setting of metabolic acidosis is to hyperventilate. CO_2 is a volatile acid, and the lungs can rapidly eliminate this acid from the body in an attempt to bring the pH closer to normal. In a patient with a HCO_3 of 4 mEq/L, for example, the $PaCO_2$ will be 14-15 mm Hg if there's appropriate respiratory compensation. This requires a very high minute ventilation to accomplish.

It is very difficult to set the ventilator to provide a high minute ventilation, even if you set the rate to be 30-35 and the tidal volume to be 800-1000 mL. Patients with severe metabolic acidosis will often breathe in when the vent is trying to breathe out, and vice versa— this leads to significant patient-ventilator dyssynchrony and alarming of the machine. More consequentially, the volume and pressure alarms that are normally helpful will actually work against the patient by limiting the minute ventilation that can occur.

Consider the aforementioned example—a patient who has a pH of 6.88 and a HCO_3 of 4 needs a $PaCO_2$ of 14-15. If he's intubated and sedated, and the vent settings are put in the "usual" range, his $PaCO_2$ may rise to 25-30. In the setting of severe acidemia, this increase in CO_2 will cause his pH to fall to 6.6 or so, which will most likely lead to a cardiac arrest.

The best way to deal with this situation is to let the patient's naturally high respiratory drive work in his favor.

1. Use the *bare minimum* of sedation to intubate and avoid neuromuscular blockers <u>entirely</u>.
2. Set the vent mode to be Pressure Support Ventilation.
3. CPAP (a.k.a. PEEP) 5-10 cm H_2O, depending on the degree of hypoxemia
4. Pressure Support (PS) of 10-15 cm H_2O. Adjust if needed to allow the patient to breathe comfortably; most of the time, 10 cm is enough PS.
5. Allow the patient to have a high minute ventilation—it may be 18-25 L/min or higher. Don't be alarmed to see him pull spontaneous volumes of 1000-2000 mL. The high minute ventilation will keep the pH up while the cause of the metabolic acidosis is being treated.

Key Concepts for Other Clinical Situations

- The left ventricle likes PEEP—increasing the intrathoracic pressure lowers preload and afterload, which is beneficial in acute cardiac failure due to left ventricular dysfunction (either systolic or diastolic).
- The right ventricle, on the other hand, doesn't care for PEEP very much. Increased intrathoracic pressure can increase pulmonary vascular pressures and stress the thin-walled RV. In situations where RV failure is present (massive pulmonary embolism, worsening pulmonary hypertension), use more FiO_2 and less PEEP (ideally 10 cm or less) to maintain oxygenation.
- When there is acute brain injury, be it from stroke, hemorrhage, trauma, or something else, the priority with mechanical ventilation is the maintenance of adequate oxygenation. Aim for an SpO_2 of 94-98% and a PaO_2 of 80-100 mm Hg. PEEP may increase the intracranial pressure, but it seems to be significant only when the PEEP is 15 or higher. Hypoxemia, on the other hand, definitely increases intracranial pressure. Therefore, use what it takes to maintain adequate cerebral oxygenation.
- Hyperventilation ($PaCO_2 < 32$) lowers intracranial pressure, but it works by causing cerebral vasoconstriction. In other words, it works by making the brain ischemic. This may be helpful if a patient is about to herniate, and you need 5 minutes to get the mannitol in or 10 minutes to get to the OR. Prolonged hyperventilation, on the other hand, worsens brain ischemia and has no lasting effect on intracranial hypertension. Aim for a normal (35-40) $PaCO_2$.

Noninvasive Positive Pressure Ventilation

NIPPV refers to positive pressure ventilation using a mask or helmet, not an endotracheal tube. It can provide a continuous positive airway pressure (CPAP) or both an inspiratory and expiratory pressure (BiPAP).

CPAP is used to treat obstructive sleep apnea. In the acute setting, it's also useful for cardiogenic pulmonary edema. The positive pressure helps open flooded alveoli; improves work of breathing; and reduces cardiac preload and afterload. This provides respiratory support while you wait for your other interventions to work (diuresis, afterload reduction).

Typical CPAP settings are between **5 and 10 cm H₂O.** If a patient has obstructive sleep apnea, a higher pressure may be needed as a "pneumatic splint" for the upper airway.

BiPAP uses two pressures—an expiratory pressure (EPAP), which is the same as CPAP; and an inspiratory pressure (IPAP), which is analogous to Pressure Support on the ventilator. BiPAP is useful when a patient needs both positive airway pressure and some inspiratory assistance. Clinical situations where BiPAP is preferred include obesity hypoventilation syndrome, laryngeal edema, congestive heart failure, and a COPD exacerbation with hypercapnia.

The EPAP should be set in the same way you set PEEP. A patient with considerable pulmonary edema may need an EPAP of 8-10 cm H_2O, and a patient with a large neck and obstructive sleep apnea may need an EPAP of 10-12 to splint the airway. Someone with COPD, on the other hand, has the opposite problem—there's hyperinflation of alveoli and nothing that needs to be splinted open. Use the lowest EPAP setting (typically 2-4).

The IPAP provides the inspiratory boost when the patient triggers the breath. For example, a BiPAP setting of 18/10 means that the machine goes from an expiratory pressure of 10 to a total pressure of 18 during inspiration. This may be different from PSV on the ventilator—in PSV, the PS is added to the CPAP. You can adjust the IPAP to provide effective alveolar ventilation. This doesn't require getting a blood gas every hour. Base your adjustments on how the patient looks. Many BiPAP machines will report a tidal volume, but keep in mind the leaks around the mask make this inaccurate.

A good starting point for BiPAP is 10/5 (IPAP 10, EPAP 5). If the patient is hypercapnic he may need more of a boost—12 or 15/5. If he has considerable pulmonary edema and hypoxemia, then a setting of 18/10 would be appropriate. The inspiratory assistance is the difference between the IPAP and EPAP—the boost during the patient's breath is the same for BiPAP settings of 15/5 and 20/10. 10 cm H_2O pressure is applied to the EPAP during inspiration.

NIPPV requires that the patient be capable of breathing on his own (there's no set rate) and have protective airway reflexes. An obtunded patient with secretions pooling in his throat is not an ideal BiPAP candidate. If you do put a patient on BiPAP, be sure to reassess him in 30-60 minutes to see if he's improving. If he's not, consider moving on to intubation and mechanical ventilation.

Tidal Volume Chart—Females

Height (ft/in)	4 mL/kg PBW	6 mL/kg PBW	8 mL/kg PBW
5' 0	182	273	364
5' 1	191	287	382
5' 2	200	301	401
5' 3	210	314	419
5' 4	219	328	438
5' 5	228	342	456
5' 6	237	356	474
5' 7	246	370	493
5' 8	256	383	511
5' 9	265	397	530
5' 10	274	411	548
5' 11	283	425	566
6' 0	292	439	585
6' 1	302	452	603
6' 2	311	466	622
6' 3	320	480	640
6' 4	329	494	658
6' 5	338	508	677
6' 6	348	521	695
6' 7	357	535	714
6' 8	366	549	732
6' 9	375	563	750
6' 10	384	577	769
6' 11	394	590	787
7' 0	403	604	806

Tidal Volume Chart—Males

Height (ft/in)	4 mL/kg PBW	6 mL/kg PBW	8 mL/kg PBW
5' 0	200	300	400
5' 1	209	314	418
5' 2	218	328	437
5' 3	228	341	455
5' 4	237	355	474
5' 5	246	369	492
5' 6	255	383	510
5' 7	264	397	529
5' 8	274	410	547
5' 9	283	424	566
5' 10	292	438	584
5' 11	301	452	602
6' 0	310	466	621
6' 1	320	479	639
6' 2	329	493	658
6' 3	338	507	676
6' 4	347	521	694
6' 5	356	535	713
6' 6	366	548	731
6' 7	375	562	750
6' 8	384	576	768
6' 9	393	590	786
6' 10	402	604	805
6' 11	412	617	823
7' 0	421	631	842

Easy PEEP Table

Degree of ARDS	PaO$_2$/FiO$_2$ Ratio	PEEP
Mild	201-300	5-10 cm H$_2$O
Moderate	101-200	10-15 cm H$_2$O
Severe	≤ 100	15-20 cm H$_2$O

ARDSNet Low PEEP Table

FiO$_2$	PEEP
30%	5
40%	5
40%	8
50%	8
50%	10
60%	10
70%	10
70%	12
70%	14
80%	14
90%	14
90%	16
90%	18
100%	18
100%	20
100%	22
100%	24

ARDSNet High PEEP Table

FiO$_2$	PEEP
30%	5
30%	8
30%	10
30%	12
30%	14
40%	14
40%	16
50%	16
50%	18
50%	20
60%	20
70%	20
80%	20
80%	22
90%	22
100%	22
100%	24

Quick Ventilator Troubleshooting

Problem: Gas Exchange Abnormalities

These are ways to adjust the ventilator based on the arterial blood gas. Obviously, the patient's condition should dictate what's done. The adjustments are in order of preference.

PaO_2 Too Low
- Assist-Control, SIMV: increase PEEP, increase FiO_2
- APRV: increase P_{HIGH}, increase T_{HIGH}, increase FiO_2

$PaCO_2$ Too High
- Volume Assist-Control or SIMV: increase rate, increase tidal volume
- Pressure Assist-Control or SIMV: increase rate, increase driving pressure
- APRV: increase the gradient between P_{HIGH} and P_{LOW}, decrease T_{HIGH}, increase T_{LOW}

$PaCO_2$ Too Low
- Volume Assist-Control or SIMV: decrease rate, lower tidal volume
- Pressure Assist-Control or SIMV: decrease rate, lower driving pressure
- APRV: increase T_{HIGH}, lower P_{HIGH}, decrease T_{LOW}

59

Ventilator Pressures and Monitors

These are problems that you'll be called about. As always, the first thing you should do is examine the patient. Remember your ABCs and use this guide to help you figure out what's wrong.

Problem: High Peak Airway (P_{AW}) Pressure

Your first step should be to perform an inspiratory pause and measure the plateau pressure (P_{PLAT}). The plateau pressure represents the alveolar pressure, while the peak pressure is a combination of the alveolar pressure and airway resistance.

High P_{AW}, Low P_{PLAT}—this means the problem is high airway resistance.
- Kinked endotracheal tube—unkink the tube
- Mucus plugging—pass a suction catheter
- Bronchospasm—inhaled bronchodilators
- Too narrow of an endotracheal tube—change the tube, or accept higher P_{AW}

High P_{AW}, High P_{PLAT}—this means the problem is in the lungs.
- Mainstem intubation—pull the endotracheal tube back into the trachea
- Atelectasis of a lobe or lung—chest percussion, or bronchoscopy to open up the airway
- Pulmonary edema—diuretics or inotropes
- ARDS—use a lower tidal volume, higher PEEP strategy
- Pneumothorax—chest tube

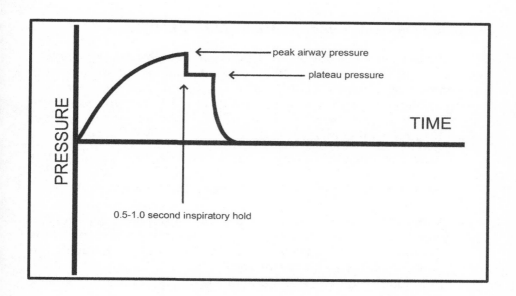

The plateau pressure represents the equilibration of pressures throughout the lungs when flow is stopped. This is the best assessment of the alveolar pressure. The *difference* between the peak airway pressure and the plateau pressure represents the resistance of the conducting airways. This is normally < 5 cm H_2O. An increase in the gradient between the peak and plateau pressures indicates high airway resistance.

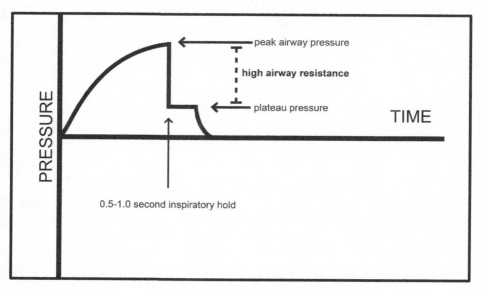

Problem: Dynamic Hyperinflation (Auto-PEEP)

This is usually due to inadequate time for exhalation. High airway resistance (bronchospasm, COPD, mucus plugging) makes it worse. On exam, the patient's abdominal muscles will contract forcefully during exhalation. Neck veins may be distended, and you may hear loud wheezing. The ventilator's expiratory flow waveform will not return to the baseline of zero flow.

- Lower the ventilator rate, usually between 10-14 breaths per minute
- Shorten the inspiratory time to keep the I:E ratio in the 1:3 – 1:5 range
- Keep the tidal volume in the 6-8 mL/kg range—a higher tidal volume will often slow the patient's spontaneous respirations
- Increase the inspiratory flow to 60-80 liters per minute if the patient seems to be "air hungry"
- Adequate sedation with narcotics will help blunt a tachypneic response
- Treat bronchospasm with inhaled bronchodilators and systemic steroids

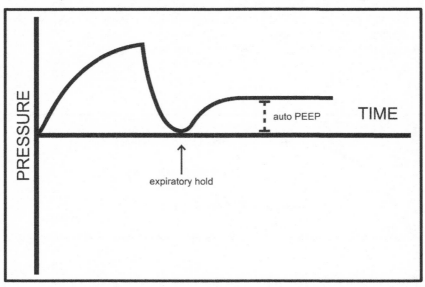

The end-expiratory pressure represents the equilibration of pressures throughout the lungs when flow is stopped. This is the best assessment of the alveolar pressure. If the pressure at end-expiration exceeds the applied (set by the machine) PEEP, then there is autoPEEP present. Normally, there should be no difference between the end-expiratory pressure and the set PEEP.

Problem: Sudden Drop in SpO$_2$

New or worsening hypoxemia is always cause for alarm. The first step is to exclude mechanical problems or tube displacement.

- Disconnect the patient from the ventilator and bag him
- Make sure the tube is in place (use either color-change or waveform capnometry if there's any doubt about the tube) and that breath sounds are present and equal
- Obtain an arterial blood gas
- Chest X-ray—this will show you worsening infiltrates, pneumothorax, pulmonary edema, atelectasis, or new effusions
- Always consider pulmonary embolism as a cause for new hypoxemia in an ICU patient, and have a low threshold for diagnostic studies
- Absent breath sounds on one side—pull the endotracheal tube back a few centimeters
- Absent breath sounds on one side, even with the tube in the right place—think pneumothorax, or mucus plugging with complete atelectasis of the lung
- Tension pneumothorax should be suspected if breath sounds are absent on one side and if the patient is hypotensive. Distended neck veins and tracheal shift away from the affected side are supportive but not always seen. The treatment is immediate needle decompression and placement of a chest tube.

Problem: Fighting the Ventilator

Before sedating or paralyzing a patient for "fighting the ventilator," you should always check **TSS**—**T**ube, **S**ounds, **S**ats. Make sure that the endotracheal tube is in place and not obstructed, that breath sounds are present and equal, and that the patient is not hypoxemic. Other things you should look for are:

- Dynamic hyperinflation (see above for how to treat this)
- Untreated pain, especially in trauma and surgical patients
- Make sure the vent is providing an adequate rate and tidal volume
- Switch to assist-control ventilation if the patient is getting fatigued
- Search for other causes of distress—cardiac ischemia, fever, abdominal distension, neurologic deterioration, etc.

Problem: Change in End-Tidal CO₂

First, look at the waveform. If there is no waveform, it means one of three things:
- The endotracheal or tracheostomy tube is not in the trachea
- The tube is completely occluded
- The $ETCO_2$ sensor is faulty

Obviously, the first two are serious emergencies and should be dealt with immediately. The third is diagnosed only after ruling out the first two.

If the waveform is present, then look at the $ETCO_2$ value. With a significant change in the $ETCO_2$, an arterial blood gas should be obtained as well to see what the $PaCO_2$ is.

Rising $ETCO_2$ and $PaCO_2$—this indicates either increased CO_2 production or alveolar hypoventilation.
- Fever
- Malignant hyperthermia
- Thyrotoxicosis
- Suppressed respiratory drive without a sufficient ventilator backup rate

Falling $ETCO_2$ with unchanged or rising $PaCO_2$—the widening gradient between the two suggests an increase in dead space ventilation.
- Pulmonary embolism
- Falling cardiac output (cardiogenic or hypovolemic shock)
- Dynamic hyperinflation with autoPEEP

Falling $ETCO_2$ and falling $PaCO_2$—indicates an increase in alveolar ventilation.

- Pain
- Agitation
- Fever
- Sepsis

Critical Care Airway Management Flowchart*

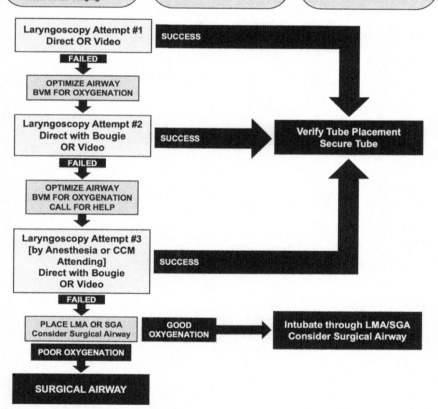

* IMPORTANT—this assumes you know what you're doing or are in the company of someone who does. Airways can go bad in a *hurry* so always be sure you have support immediately available.

Neurocritical Care

What You Need To Survive

Acute brain injury is common in the ICU. Many times, it's due to something else going on with the patient—septic encephalopathy, delirium, hypotension, electrolyte imbalance, etc. In these cases, correcting the cause usually improves brain function. Sometimes, the patient is in the ICU because of direct injury to the brain. This can usually be divided into one of two camps— "toxic-metabolic" injury or "structural" injury. Structural brain injury can be from trauma, edema, spontaneous hemorrhage, or vascular occlusion. This section covers:

- Top priorities of neurocritical care
- Blood pressure goals for different neurologic conditions
- Glasgow Coma Score
- Sedatives used in the ICU
- Richmond Agitation-Sedation Scale
- Management of intracranial hypertension
- An overview of how a ventriculostomy drain works
- Common sodium-related disorders seen in neurocritical care

Four Graphs That Illustrate the Priorities of Neurocritical Care

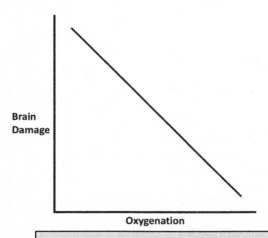

Brain Damage
Oxygenation

Avoiding hypoxemia is one of the most important things you can do in patients with CNS injury. There's not a whole lot of evidence that defines the "critical threshold" of oxygen tension in the brain, but it makes sense to keep the patient well-oxygenated.

Try to keep the SpO$_2$ at least 95% and the PaO$_2$ at least 90 mm Hg.

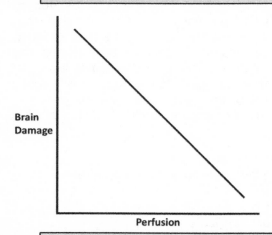

Brain Damage
Perfusion

Perfusion goes hand in hand with oxygenation. CNS autoregulation is lost during acute brain injury, so it's essential to maintain adequate blood flow of oxygenated blood.

Aim to keep the SBP at least 90, and ideally > 100. If you have an ICP monitor, keep the cerebral perfusion pressure 60-80.

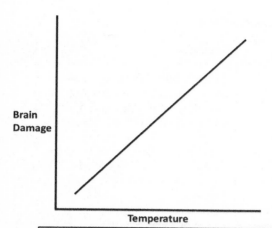

Brain Damage / Temperature

Every degree C° above normal increases cerebral metabolic oxygen consumption by 6-7%. Normally this is well-tolerated; however, with acute brain injury, this can be deleterious. Aggressive antipyretics and cooling measures should be used.

Keep the patient normothermic. Induced hypothermia may be necessary in some situations.

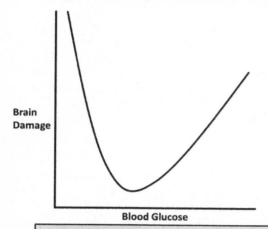

Brain Damage / Blood Glucose

Hypoglycemia is very dangerous—brain tissue has very few glycogen stores and depends on a continuous supply of either glucose or ketones for energy. Hyperglycemia, especially when the glucose exceeds 400 mg/dL, is also associated with worse outcomes.

Aim for a blood glucose in the 100-200 mg/dL range. This should keep the patient from becoming hypoglycemic yet maintain adequate glycemic control.

Blood Pressure Goals in Neurocritical Care

Condition	Target BP	Rationale
Subarachnoid Hemorrhage	MAP 70-90 SBP 100-150	Systolic blood pressure spikes above 150 increase the risk of rerupture of the aneurysm, which carries a 75% risk of mortality.
Intracerebral Hemorrhage	MAP 100-120 SBP 120-160	Cerebral perfusion needs to be maintained, but the blood pressure should be lowered rapidly to prevent expansion of the hematoma.
Hypertensive Encephalopathy	Reduction of the MAP by 25% over 1 hour	Rapid lowering of the blood pressure beyond 25% of the initial MAP may cause cerebral ischemia and other end-organ damage.
Acute Ischemic Stroke	Don't lower the blood pressure unless the SBP exceeds 220 or the DBP exceeds 120, **unless thrombolytics have been given or a thrombectomy has been performed.**	After an ischemic stroke, a "penumbra" of viable, but threatened, brain tissue exists around the infarcted area. This penumbra depends on collateral circulation and adequate perfusion, and dropping the blood pressure can lead to death of this tissue. So, while the temptation to lower the BP is there, RESIST!
Post-Thrombolysis for Stroke	MAP 100-130 SBP 140-180 DBP < 105	After tPA, the balance is between adequate perfusion of the penumbra and the risk of hemorrhage with higher blood pressures.

So, now that you've decided to lower the blood pressure, what drug do you use? Again, much of this depends on the clinical situation. Here are some drugs that are commonly used in neurocritical care.

Drug	Dose	Mechanism, Pros and Cons
Nicardipine	5-15 mg/hr infusion	Calcium channel blocker with no suppression of the AV node; acts as a cerebral arterial vasodilator. Very titratable with few side effects and preferred for most neurocritical care patients.
Labetalol	10-20 mg IV PRN 0.5-2.0 mg/min infusion	Combined alpha and beta receptor blocker; especially useful in hyperadrenergic conditions (cocaine intoxication, thyrotoxicosis). Can cause bradycardia and bronchospasm.
Hydralazine	10 mg IV q4h	Reduces afterload Can cause tachycardia

Glasgow Coma Score (GCS)

Component	Response	Score
Eye Opening	Spontaneously	4
	To voice	3
	To noxious stimuli	2
	No response	1
Verbal Response	Coherent, fluent speech	5
	Confused speech	4
	Inappropriate words	3
	Moans and groans	2
	No response	1
Motor Response	Follows directions	6
	Localizes to noxious stimuli	5
	Withdrawal from noxious stimuli	4
	Decorticate (flexor) posturing	3
	Decerebrate (extensor) posturing	2
	No response	1
Total Score	Best response	15
	Mild brain injury	13-15
	Moderate brain injury	9-12
	Severe brain injury	3-8

Intubated patients cannot speak, so assign the value of T for the verbal response. The best response would be 10T, and the worst response is 2T.

Typical Sedatives and Analgesics in the ICU

Continuous Infusions

- Propofol 10-50 mcg/kg/min
- Midazolam 1-20 mg/hr
- Dexmedetomidine 0.2-1.7 mcg/kg/hr
- Fentanyl 25-200 mcg/hr

As-Needed Medications

- Lorazepam 1-4 mg IV every 1-4 hours
- Fentanyl 25-50 mcg IV every 1-2 hours
- Haloperidol 2-5 mg IV every 4-6 hours
- Olanzapine 10 mg IM every 6 hours

Sedation is generally titrated toward a sedation score, such as a RASS of 0 to -1.

Richmond Agitation-Sedation Scale (RASS)

Term	Description	Score
Combative	Combative, violent, danger to staff	+4
Very Agitated	Aggressive, pulling tubes and lines	+3
Agitated	Frequent movement, bucking the ventilator	+2
Restless	Vigorous movement but not aggressive	+1
Alert, Calm	Responsive and calm	0
Drowsy	Responds to voice and maintains at least 10 seconds of eye contact	-1
Light Sedation	Responds to voice but maintains less than 10 seconds of eye contact	-2
Moderate Sedation	Moves or opens eyes to voice but makes no eye contact	-3
Deep Sedation	Moves or opens eyes to physical stimulation but not voice	-4
Unarousable	No response to voice or physical stimulation	-5

Intracranial Hypertension

Intracranial pressure (ICP) can be measured by a pressure transducer inserted into the brain, an epidural pressure sensor (also known as a bolt), or by a catheter inserted into either the lateral cerebral ventricle (ventriculostomy) or the lumbar thecal sac (lumbar drain). Ventriculostomy is the most common method and the most accurate. In addition to measuring the ICP, the ventriculostomy can also be used to drain CSF when the ICP is too high.

Parenchymal and epidural pressure sensors are useful when a ventriculostomy cannot be inserted, but their accuracy fades over time. They also have no therapeutic benefit, as they cannot be used to drain CSF.

Lumbar drains are inserted when there is good communication between the brain and spinal CSF. If there is brain mass effect or an obstruction to flow, lowering the lumbar CSF pressure could lead to brain herniation.

The ICP is considered elevated when it exceeds 10 mm Hg. The more important consideration is the cerebral perfusion pressure (CPP), which is calculated by subtracting the ICP from the mean arterial pressure:

$$CPP = MAP - ICP$$

CPP less than 50 can lead to dangerous cerebral ischemia. CPP above 120 can lead to cerebral edema. Since injured brain tissue loses a great deal of its autoregulation, it makes sense to target a CPP of 60-80 to ensure adequate cerebral perfusion. This may require norepinephrine or other vasopressors even if the blood pressure is above the typical MAP of 65.

If the ICP exceeds 20 mm Hg it generally needs rapid correction.

Measures To Control Intracranial Hypertension

FIRST LINE INTERVENTIONS	
Ensure adequate oxygenation—PaO_2 90-100, SaO_2 95-98%	Sufficiently oxygenate the vulnerable CNS
Keep $PaCO_2$ 35-40, pH 7.35-7.45	Hypercapnia can cause cerebral vasodilation and increase ICP
Increase MAP to keep CPP > 60, using IV fluids and vasopressors	Ensure adequate cerebral perfusion
Sedation and analgesia	Goal RASS -1 to -2 to reduce cerebral oxygen demands
Treat fever	Every °C above 37 increases cerebral metabolic oxygen consumption by 6-7%
Head of bed elevation	30-40 degrees to facilitate venous drainage
CSF drainage if ventriculostomy is present	Drain 5-10 mL CSF
SECOND LINE INTERVENTIONS	
Mild hyperventilation—$PaCO_2$ 30-35, pH 7.40-7.45	Mild hyperventilation causes cerebral vasoconstriction, lowering the ICP. Caution: excessive hyperventilation can cause cerebral ischemia. Prolonged hyperventilation loses its effectiveness over time.
Osmotherapy: 3% saline (bolus and infusion)	Bolus 2 mL/kg, followed by infusion of 0.5 mL/kg/hr. Titrate to keep the serum sodium 145-155. Consider adding furosemide in patients with cardiac or renal disease.

Osmotherapy: Mannitol	0.25-1.0 g/kg bolus. This can be repeated every 4-6 hours but loses its effectiveness over time. Mannitol is a diuretic and should be used with caution if the patient is hypovolemic.
THIRD LINE INTERVENTIONS	
Pharmacotherapy: Propofol or pentobarbital coma	Propofol 50-80 mcg/kg/min Pentobarbital 10 mg/kg over 60 minutes, then 5 mg/kg/hr for 3 hours, then 1-5 mg/kg/hr
Pharmacotherapy: Neuromuscular blockade	Rocuronium or cisatracurium infusion Requires sedation to RASS -4 to -5 as well
Surgical Therapy: Decompressive craniectomy Temporal lobectomy	More useful with unilateral pathology
Therapeutic Hypothermia	Consider cooling to 32-34°C for refractory intracranial hypertension not amenable to surgery

Simplified Ventriculostomy Diagram

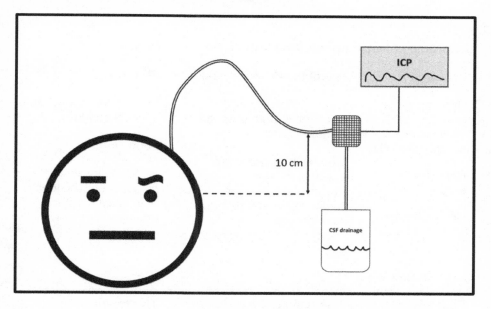

The ventriculostomy catheter is inserted in the patient's right lateral ventricle. The transducer's zero point is level with the patient's midbrain (dashed line). The drain is then positioned at a selected height above midbrain—in this case, 10 cm. This means that if the ICP exceeds 10 cm H_2O pressure, CSF will flow through the tubing and into the drainage bag.

The ventriculostomy catheter can also be transduced on a standard pressure monitor. To do this, the drainage bag is "clamped" so no CSF can drain. The ICP is then displayed on the monitor screen. An appropriate ICP waveform looks like an arterial waveform, with the peak coinciding with the systolic blood pressure.

Note that while the height of the drain is often set in cm H_2O pressure, blood pressure and the transduced ICP are in mm Hg. 1 cm H_2O = 0.76 mm Hg. In this example, the ICP must exceed 10 cm H_2O, or 7.6 mm Hg, for CSF to drain. This is important because cerebral perfusion pressure (CPP) is calculated by subtracting the ICP from the patient's mean arterial pressure (MAP). Since MAP is measured in mm Hg, ICP must be as well.

Common Sodium Disorders in Neurocritical Care

Syndrome of Inappropriate Antidiuretic Hormone (SIADH)

Features	Associated Conditions	Treatment
Hyponatremia Urine osmolality > serum osmolality Restricted urine output Uric acid low	Seen with many CNS conditions, both traumatic and nontraumatic Can also be seen with congestive heart failure, chronic lung disease, malignancy, and related to medications	Free water restriction to 1500 mL/day Loop diuretics Hypertonic saline in conjunction with loop diuretics if cerebral edema is present

Cerebral Salt Wasting

Features	Associated Conditions	Treatment
Hyponatremia Urine osmolality > serum osmolality High urine output; can lead to volume depletion Uric acid normal or high	Almost always seen with aneurysmal subarachnoid hemorrhage	Hypertonic saline, using a solution that has a higher tonicity than the urine osmolality— 1.8% saline: 616 mEq/L 3% saline: 1026 mEq/L Avoid diuretics!

Central Diabetes Insipidus

Features	Associated Conditions	Treatment
Hypernatremia Polyuria Urine osmolality much lower than serum osmolality Low urine specific gravity (looks almost like water)	Cerebral anoxia Traumatic brain injury Injury to the posterior pituitary gland (e.g., surgery for craniopharyngioma)	DDAVP 1 mcg IV q6h LR @ 1-1.5 mL/kg/hr to prevent volume depletion Replace all urinary losses *in excess of 200 mL/hr* with D5W

Renal

What To Know On Rounds

- Urine output (either the amount, if measured, or the frequency of voiding)
- Net ultrafiltration rate (if on CRRT)
- Fluid balance (accurate daily weights are the best; a 24-hour fluid balance is helpful; the total fluid balance is nice but is frequently inaccurate). This can also be estimated based on edema, ascites, pleural effusions, etc.
- Renal indices (BUN, creatinine, GFR)
- Any fluid deficits that need correcting
- Is the patient's intrinsic renal function adequate, or does he need help?
    - Diuretics?
    - Renal replacement therapy?

What You Need To Know To Survive

Renal function can be adversely affected by many critical illnesses and injuries. Support of renal function focuses on maintenance of fluid status and correction of electrolytes. Many times, renal function can be an indicator of the patient's overall status—worsening renal function is a sign of developing sepsis, worsening cardiac function, or hemorrhage, while improving renal function is often one of the first signs of recovery. This section covers:

- Diagnostic criteria for acute kidney injury
- Workup for acute kidney injury
- Sodium bicarbonate treatment for acidosis
- Diuretic therapy
- Vascular access options for renal replacement therapy
- An overview of continuous renal replacement therapy
- Guidelines for intravenous fluids and correcting deficits

Typical "acceptable" urine output is at least 0.3-0.5 mL/kg/hr (using ideal body weight).

Oliguria is usually defined as < 500 mL of urine in a 24-hour period.

Acute kidney injury (AKI) is typically when the creatinine rises by 0.5 mg/dL or is at least 1.5 times the baseline (if known). Acute renal failure (ARF) is a synonymous term but is used more often when the patient ends up needing renal replacement therapy (RRT).

KDIGO Criteria for AKI Staging

Stage	Creatinine Criteria	Urine Output Criteria
0	1.4 × baseline or less	0.5 mL/kg/hr or more
1	1.5-1.9 × baseline **or** increased by > 0.3 mg/dL	< 0.5 mL/kg/hr for 6-12 hours
2	2.0-2.9 × baseline	< 0.5 mL/kg/hr for > 12 hours
3	> 3 × baseline **or** > 4 mg/dL **or** initiation of RRT	< 0.3 mL/kg/hr for > 24 hours **or** anuria > 12 hours

The stage is generally given to the worst feature (creatinine or urine output). The need for renal replacement therapy is more correlated with the urine output criteria. The mortality risk is more correlated by the combination of the two.

Initial Testing For Acute Kidney Injury

Rule out urinary obstruction

- Bladder outlet obstruction is a common cause of anuria. Placing a Foley catheter can be both diagnostic and therapeutic and will help you follow the response to therapy.
- Renal ultrasound or CT should be done to make sure there isn't hydronephrosis. If there is an obstruction of the ureters, urologic consultation is in order.

Review the chart
- Look for inciting events—periods of hypotension in particular, but also things like new medications (especially NSAIDs, ACE-inhibitors, and antibiotics), IV contrast administration, or recent endovascular procedures (cholesterol emboli).
- Having previous lab data is helpful to decide if this is all AKI or if the patient has chronic kidney disease.

Lab testing
- Serum electrolytes, including $Ca/Mg/PO_4$; be sure to see if the anion gap is elevated
- Serum osmolarity if there's concern for toxic alcohol ingestion
- Creatinine kinase
- Urinalysis with microscopy
- Therapeutic drug levels if indicated (vancomycin, aminoglycosides, acetaminophen, salicylate)
- Uric acid if there's concern for tumor lysis syndrome
- Generally unhelpful labs
  - Fractional excretion of sodium or urea
  - Urine eosinophils

Treatment of Acute Kidney Injury

Ensure euvolemia, either by physical exam or with bedside ultrasound. A fluid bolus is often given to see whether there's a response—isotonic fluids (0.9% saline, Lactated Ringers, Plasmalyte) are best for this. Keep in mind that with the volume of fluids needed for sedatives, antibiotics, vasopressors, and other medications, **it is unusual for anyone to be volume-depleted after 24 hours in the ICU**.

Kidneys work best when the intravascular volume is normal. Both hypo- and hypervolemia can lead to acute kidney injury.

Avoid nephrotoxic medications like aminoglycosides, NSAIDs, and ACE-inhibitors. Consultation with a critical care pharmacist to renally adjust medication doses is very helpful.

Most students are taught the "AEIOU" mnemonic for when to initiate dialysis—*acidosis*, *electrolyte* disturbance, *intoxication*, volume *overload*, and *uremic* symptoms. In the ICU, this can be simplified even further: refractory acidosis, life-threatening hyperkalemia, and volume overload.

- Refractory acidosis means that despite aggressive medical therapy, the patient continues to have a pH less than 7.2 with respiratory or hemodynamic compromise. Before initiating dialysis, treatment with sodium bicarbonate should be initiated (boluses and an infusion). Acidemia due to ketoacidosis is easily treated with insulin (for DKA) and dextrose (for starvation or alcoholic ketoacidosis) and renal replacement therapy is seldom necessary. Most intoxications that require urgent RRT also cause a metabolic acidosis—iron, aspirin, methanol, and ethylene glycol are common ones.

- Hyperkalemia is considered life-threatening whenever there are ECG changes associated with it and it should be treated aggressively. Hyperkalemia and acidemia often go hand in hand and boluses of sodium bicarbonate will often fix the issue; however, if there is associated renal failure, RRT is usually needed.

- Volume overload in the setting of oliguric renal failure that is refractory to diuretic therapy often warrants RRT. A trial of diuresis to convert oliguric to non-oliguric renal failure is worthwhile and may save the patient a dialysis catheter.

Sodium bicarbonate

Bolus Therapy
- One ampule of 8.4% sodium bicarbonate is 50 mEq/50 mL
- For severe metabolic acidosis (pH < 7.2 with associated shock), give sodium bicarbonate using this formula: 0.3 × weight (kg) × base deficit = mEq needed [round to the nearest multiple of 50 mEq]

Infusion Therapy
- For mild-to-moderate metabolic acidosis (pH > 7.2), mix 50-100 mEq of sodium bicarbonate in one liter of either D5W or sterile water. Infuse at a rate of 1-1.5 mL/kg/hr. Keeping the solution hypotonic helps avoid sodium overload.
- For more severe metabolic acidosis (pH < 7.2), mix 150 mEq of sodium bicarbonate in one liter of D5W or sterile water. Infuse at a rate of 1-1.5 mL/kg/hr. This isotonic fluid has more bicarbonate but also more sodium, so pulmonary edema is a risk.

- For severe metabolic acidosis where aggressive correction is necessary (shock, cardiac failure, prolonged QRS interval, hyperkalemia), mix a solution of 150 mEq sodium bicarbonate in 150 mL sterile water. This is hypertonic and must be given through a central venous line. Infuse at a rate of 10-50 mL/hr, depending on the severity of the acidemia. This can cause significant hypernatremia, so check electrolytes frequently.

Diuretics

Diuretics can be used to challenge the kidneys to convert oliguria to nonoliguria, or when the total body volume is too high.

Hypervolemia can actually worsen renal function, which may not be immediately intuitive. If the central venous pressure is elevated, then the perfusion pressure gradient in the kidney will be reduced, thereby reducing glomerular filtration. In addition, volume excess can increase the interstitial pressure within the kidney itself (kind of like a mini compartment syndrome), which also reduces renal function.

Converting oliguric renal failure to nonoliguric has not been clearly demonstrated to reduce mortality; however, it does make fluid management much easier and keeps the patient from having to receive dialysis (which is an important goal in itself). Additionally, several studies have not shown a survival benefit to earlier initiation of RRT, so it doesn't seem to be harmful to give a trial of diuretics.

Diuretic Tips

- 20-40 × serum creatinine (for a creatinine of 2.5 mg/dL, 50-100 mg furosemide) can be given as a bolus. Remember that diuresis depends on getting an adequate amount of the drug to the receptors in the Loop of Henle (LoH)—therefore, if the response isn't adequate (typically < 200 mL urine 1-2 hours after the bolus), increase the dose of furosemide. If 80 mg furosemide only produced 70 mL urine, dosing 80 mg every 6 hours won't lead to a suitable diuresis since the drug never sufficiently saturates the receptors.

- If the response to the furosemide bolus was adequate but the overall diuresis isn't enough, increase the frequency of drug dosing. Once the receptors in the LoH are saturated, increasing the dose won't add much (e.g., if 80 mg furosemide produced 350 mL of urine, increasing to 160 mg won't double the output). Increasing the frequency is the way to get more fluid off of the patient.

- An alternative to intermittent furosemide dosing is to give a bolus, followed by an infusion of 5-20 mg/hr. The initial bolus dose saturates the LoH receptors, and the infusion keeps them saturated. The infusion can be titrated to maintain a urine output of 1-2 mL/kg/hr. The infusion also causes less episodic hypotension than intermittent dosing.

- If the patient's hemodynamics are tenuous, or if he has significant hypoproteinemia (albumin < 2.5 g/dL), then albumin can be added to the diuretic regimen. Typically, 12.5 g of 25% albumin is given IV every 6 hours, along with either a furosemide infusion or furosemide dosed every 6 hours. If you're using intermittent diuretic dosing, give the furosemide 30 minutes after the albumin. The hyperoncotic albumin solution (theoretically) pulls the water from the extravascular space and the diuretic helps the kidney push it out of the body.

- There is some data that other loop diuretics like bumetanide or torsemide may work better than furosemide in certain situations like cardiac failure or hypoproteinemia. Furosemide is still the most commonly available and commonly used loop diuretic. If you choose to use one of the other agents, adjust the dosing and frequency accordingly.

- Loop diuretics impair the ability of the kidney to maximally concentrate the urine, which can lead to hypernatremia. Thiazide diuretics impair the ability of the kidney to maximally dilute the urine, which can lower the serum sodium. A volume-overloaded patient with hypernatremia may benefit from a thiazide diuretic if you want to lower the serum sodium concentration.

Renal Replacement Therapy

Renal replacement therapy (RRT) can be provided using either intermittent hemodialysis or continuous therapy. Continuous renal replacement therapy (CRRT) is better for patients with unstable hemodynamics. Both require vascular access, typically through a large-bore intravascular catheter.

Placement Options for Temporary Dialysis Lines

Site	Catheter length (most adults)	Comments
Right IJ	16 cm	Preferred site in most cases
Left IJ	20 cm	Preferred if the right IJ can't be used
Femoral	24 cm	This is less comfortable for the patient and more difficult for the nursing staff to keep clean. Use the femoral vein if the IJ sites aren't available or if RRT is only needed for a few days
Right subclavian	16 cm	If there is any concern that the patient will need long-term dialysis, avoid the subclavian veins if possible. Stenosis can cause issues with future AV graft placement.
Left subclavian	20 cm	

CRRT is a catchall term that includes different modalities of renal replacement therapy. In the vast majority of cases, CRRT refers to continuous venovenous hemodiafiltration (CVVHDF). It's venovenous because a dual lumen catheter is used to both pull blood from the vein and to return it to the venous system.

Hemodialysis refers to using a dialysate to remove small solutes like urea and potassium and to raise the level of the plasma bicarbonate. By passing the dialysate countercurrent to blood flow, small solutes will flow across a semipermeable membrane via a concentration gradient. Therefore, potassium will flow from the blood into the dialysate if the patient is hyperkalemic, and bicarbonate will flow from the dialysate into the blood if the patient is acidemic.

Hemofiltration involves using a pressure gradient across a semipermeable membrane to remove larger particles like plasma proteins. The proteins carry plasma water with them as they cross the membrane—this is known as "solvent drag." The fluid that is collected is known as the ultrafiltrate. Fluid can be pumped by the CRRT machine into the blood before the filter (e.g., prefilter) to increase the pressure gradient across the membrane. Isotonic fluid can also be pumped into the blood after filtration (e.g., postfilter) to replace electrolytes lost in the ultrafiltrate.

The combination of hemodialysis and hemofiltration accomplishes the function that the kidneys have lost: maintenance of electrolytes and pH, and volume removal. Modern CRRT machines combine the membranes needed for dialysis and hemofiltration into one filter, or "kidney," in the circuit.

Most critically ill patients are receiving considerable volumes of fluids, medications, and blood products. If CRRT is initiated for renal failure, it's important to know the amount of fluid being removed. The key element is the **net ultrafiltration rate**. The net UFR is the volume of ultrafiltration minus the total volume of intake, and this is calculated every hour. Think of this like the urine output. The ultrafiltration rate can be adjusted on the machine to account for the administration of PRBCs or medications to keep the net UFR in the desired range.

A patient in profound shock on multiple vasopressors may have a net UFR of zero—that is, his volume status is being kept even. If he receives 380 mL of IV fluids during the hour, the CRRT machine will be set to remove 380 mL of ultrafiltrate. On the other hand, a patient with anasarca and pulmonary edema may need a net UFR of 200 mL/hr. If he receives 380 mL of IV fluids during the hour, the machine will be adjusted to remove 580 mL of ultrafiltrate.

The net UFR goals should be determined by the critical care team and the consulting nephrologist based on the patient's hemodynamic status, pulmonary function, and total body volume status. This often involves tradeoffs—for example, if it's difficult to oxygenate despite aggressive vent settings, the net UFR may need to be higher even if it means the norepinephrine dose has to be increased. Because it's impossible to maintain precision due to changes in circuit flow and hemodynamics, the net UFR is typically given as a range like "50-100 mL/hr." While there is no maximum UFR, it generally doesn't go higher than 2-3 mL/kg/hr.

Fluid Administration Guidelines

- Volume of Distribution (VD): AKA total body water (TBW). 0.6 L/kg in men, 0.5 L/kg in women.
- Daily fluid requirement: 25-30 mL/kg/day (assuming no oral intake)
- Daily sodium requirement: 2 mEq/kg/day
- Daily potassium requirement: 1 mEq/kg/day
- Daily glucose requirement: 50-100 g/day

Simplified—D5 1/2NS with 40 mEq of KCl/L at 1 mL/kg/hr will provide just about all of a patient's daily fluid and electrolyte requirements. Most ICUs will have an electrolyte replacement protocol, so be sure to measure magnesium, calcium, and phosphorus on a regular basis and replace as needed. If you're concerned about renal function or hyperkalemia, it's OK to omit the potassium from the maintenance fluids.

The best maintenance fluid doesn't go in a vein, obviously—it goes in the gut. Establish and use enteral feeding whenever possible and forget about the IV fluids.

A few other considerations for fluid management:

- One liter of 0.9% saline (aka normal saline) has 9 grams of NaCl in it. NS at 125 mL/hr means 27 grams of salt per day.
- LR isn't much better—figure about 7.5 grams of sodium per liter.

- Just about every medication the patient is receiving IV is mixed in salt water. Sodium overload is a real thing and should be avoided if possible.*
- Urinary fluid losses are, for the most part, normal. There is no need to replace urinary output with fluid unless it's pathologic (like in central diabetes insipidus).
- GI, pancreatic, and other body fluids that are siphoned out of the patient with tubes and drains are not part of normal fluid losses. These are best replaced 1:1 with isotonic fluid like Lactated Ringer's solution.
- Plasma fluid deficits are best replaced with 1/2NS, not isotonic fluids. Isotonic fluids are, most of the time, for volume resuscitation from hypovolemia.
- Loop diuretics get rid of more water than sodium and are preferred when the patient is fluid-overloaded and has normal or low sodium levels.
- Thiazide diuretics get rid of more sodium than water and are preferred when the patient is fluid-overloaded and hypernatremic.

---

* During the initial resuscitation, it's not possible. Just remember that the patient got a lot of sodium and fluids early on and be sure to think about diuresis if he has persistent edema or pulmonary vascular congestion.

Isotonic Fluid Composition

Fluid	Key Electrolytes (mEq/L)	Comments
Lactated Ringers*	Na 130 Cl 109 Lactate† 28 K 4 Ca 1.5 Osmolarity 274 pH 6.5	Preferred resuscitation fluid in most cases Will not cause hyperkalemia or lactic acidosis‡
Normal Saline (0.9%)	Na 154 Cl 154 Osmolarity 308 pH 5.0	Useful for hypochloremic alkalosis Can worsen metabolic acidosis in large volumes
Sodium Bicarbonate	Na 150 HCO_3 150 Osmolarity 300	Not shelf-stable, must be mixed at time of use Preferred for patients with severe acidemia or hyperkalemia and hemodynamic instability
Plasmalyte-A	Na 140 Cl 98 Acetate 27 K 5 Mg 1.5 Gluconate 23 Osmolarity 294 pH 7.4	Mimics a normal blood chemistry and pH Not as available as LR or NS

---

* Known as Hartmann's solution in the UK, Australia, and elsewhere.

† Which is a <u>base</u> ion.

‡ Look it up on PubMed if you don't believe me.

Deficits

The first rule of fluids and electrolytes is that salt follows water. In other words, a patient who has fluid overload has sodium overload. A patient who has fluid depletion has sodium depletion. The sodium level is a concentration, not a measure of total body stores.

This means that a patient with cirrhosis who has ascites and pitting edema, and a sodium level of 110 mEq/L, does not need more sodium! His *total body water* is high; therefore, his *total body sodium* is also high. The hyponatremia means that he has more water than salt, but he has too much of both. The answer is not to give him more sodium—he needs a diuretic that gets rid of both salt and water, and preferentially more water than salt. Furosemide should do the trick.

Another patient has a sodium level of 158 mEq/L, dry mucous membranes, and poor skin turgor. He is dehydrated, which means that both his *total body water* and *total body sodium* are too low. He needs IV fluids and some sodium chloride. The hypernatremia indicates that he needs more water than salt, but he needs both.

Calculation of electrolyte and water deficits is important and can help guide your fluid therapy, but the first priority should be to assess the patient's total body fluid status. This is done by clinical exam, not the laboratory. Once you come up with a fluid prescription, the following formulas can help you fine-tune what the patient needs.

Free Water Deficit

- Deficit = ([measured Na − 140] × weight × VD*) / 140
- Replace the free water deficit over 48-72 hours—too rapid of correction can cause cerebral edema

Sodium Deficit

- Deficit = (140 − measured Na) × weight × VD
- Replace the sodium deficit at a rate that corrects the sodium level by 0.25-0.5 mEq/hr. Check the sodium level frequently, so you don't overshoot. Too rapid of correction can cause osmotic demyelination syndrome.

---

* Volume of distribution: 0.6 in men, 0.5 in women

Bicarbonate Deficit

- Deficit = (24 − measured HCO_3) × weight × 0.4
- This is the total body bicarbonate deficit and does not take into account other processes causing a metabolic acidosis. Treatment of the underlying cause is essential.
- Correct half the calculated deficit and reassess before giving more sodium bicarbonate. Typically, getting the HCO_3 to 16 is sufficient.
- For a severe acidosis where you want to correct things quickly, you can also use 0.3 × weight × base deficit, rounding to the nearest 50 mEq (amps of bicarb are in 50 mEq increments).

Formulas

Serum Osmolarity (predicted)

- (Na × 2) + (BUN / 2.8) + (Glucose / 18) + (Ethanol / 4.6)[*]
- A difference between the predicted and measured serum osmolarity > 15 may indicate toxic alcohol ingestion.
- Elevated lactate and ketones can also affect the measured osmolarity, so use this in the right clinical setting.

Body Fluid Volumes

- Volume of distribution (VD) = 0.6 L/kg (men); 0.5 L/kg (women)
- Intracellular fluid volume (ICF) = Vd × 0.67
- Extracellular fluid volume (ECF) = Vd × 0.33
- Interstitial volume = ECF × 0.75
- Plasma volume = ECF × 0.25

---

[*] BUN, glucose, and ethanol measured in mg/dL

Acid-Base Problem Solving

What You Need To Survive

Few things are as troublesome for students as dealing with complex acid-base disorders. Medical textbooks are usually not helpful, because they devote pages and pages to logarithmic curves, "K" factors, physiochemical properties of solutions, and the dreaded Henderson-Hasselbach equation. The good news is that you don't need any of that. This section covers:

- A 3-step method for solving acid-base problems
- Compensation rules for different disorders
- The differential diagnosis for gap- and non-gap metabolic acidosis

Step One: Determine the Primary Disorder

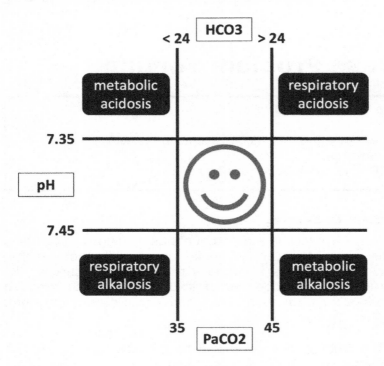

Look at the pH first. Normal pH is 7.35 to 7.45, with a dividing line at 7.40. If the pH is less than 7.35, the patient is acidemic; that is, the net charge of his bloodstream is acidic. Next, look at the $PaCO_2$. If the $PaCO_2$ is less than 40 (and usually less than 35), the problem is a metabolic acidosis. The patient is hyperventilating to rid himself of acidic carbon dioxide. If the $PaCO_2$ is greater than 40 (usually 45), the primary disorder is a respiratory acidosis. Retention of CO_2 is making the patient acidemic.

If the patient is alkalemic (his pH is greater than 7.45), a low $PaCO_2$ (less than 35) means that the primary disorder is a respiratory alkalosis. If the $PaCO_2$ is greater than 45, the primary disorder is a metabolic alkalosis and the patient is hypoventilating to control his pH.

Remember—the human body rarely, if ever, can compensate back to a normal range! That brings us to Step Two….

Step Two: Check for Compensation

Is the compensation adequate? When the primary disorder is metabolic, the patient will either hyper- or hypoventilate to try to maintain homeostasis. This is called respiratory compensation. Your next step is to determine if this compensation is adequate. If it's not, there is another disorder besides the primary one. The compensation formulas require the $PaCO_2$ and the serum HCO_3. If the HCO_3 on the serum metabolic panel and the ABG are different, go with the serum panel. It's measured, while the value on the ABG is calculated. Normal HCO_3 should be 24.

Compensation for Metabolic Acidosis:

Expected $PaCO_2 = (1.5 \times HCO_3) + 8$

For instance, if the pH is 7.22, the $PaCO_2$ is 27, and the HCO_3 is 14, we know that the primary problem is a metabolic acidosis (low pH, low $PaCO_2$). According to our compensation formula, the expected $PaCO_2$ is 29 (1.5 x 14) + 8 = 29]. Give yourself a "fudge factor" of about 2 on either side of the predicted value. Our conclusion—this patient has a <u>metabolic acidosis with appropriate respiratory compensation</u>. Try not to say that he has a "compensatory respiratory alkalosis." Alkalosis implies a pathologic process. In this case, the compensation is a perfectly normal response to acidosis.

Another example: A patient has a pH of 7.12, a $PaCO_2$ of 32, and a HCO_3 of 10. Again, the primary disorder is a metabolic acidosis. The expected $PaCO_2$, however, is 23 by the formula, and the patient's $PaCO_2$ is 32. This is higher than expected and suggests a coexistent respiratory acidosis. The diagnosis? <u>A combined respiratory and metabolic acidosis</u>. Is this a drug overdose? A septic patient with respiratory failure? Again, correlate clinically!

One more: pH 7.32, $PaCO_2$ 24, HCO_3 16. Primary disorder—metabolic acidosis. Expected $PaCO_2$—32. The $PaCO_2$ is lower than you expect, so this patient has a <u>metabolic acidosis with a coexisting respiratory alkalosis</u>.

Compensation for Metabolic Alkalosis:

Expected $PaCO_2 = (0.7 \times HCO_3) + 21$

Metabolic alkalosis is most often due to volume depletion, especially because of vomiting or NG suctioning. Hyperaldosteronism and other types of mineralocorticoid excess are other, albeit rare, causes.

An example: pH 7.52, $PaCO_2$ 42, HCO_3 30. This is a metabolic alkalosis, and the expected $PaCO_2$ is 42—this patient has a metabolic alkalosis with appropriate respiratory compensation. This could be a patient with pancreatitis who has been vomiting for three days.

What if the pH were 7.53, the HCO_3 40, and the $PaCO_2$ 60 (a CHF patient who received a 50cc bolus of sodium bicarbonate)? This is a metabolic alkalosis, but the expected $PaCO_2$ is 49. This patient has a metabolic alkalosis and a coexisting respiratory acidosis.

With respiratory disorders, you must determine if the process is acute or chronic. Generally speaking, chronic disorders have been present for 3-5 days or more, giving the kidneys time to equilibrate. Patients with chronic respiratory acidosis (emphysematous "CO_2 retainers") usually have a near-normal pH despite high $PaCO_2$ levels; clinically, they can tolerate higher levels of $PaCO_2$ without becoming obtunded. The compensation formulas are:

Compensation for Respiratory Acidosis:

- **Acute: HCO_3 rises 1 for every 10 the $PaCO_2$ rises**
- **Chronic: HCO_3 rises 3-4 for every 10 the $PaCO_2$ rises**

For instance, if a patient with emphysema has a pH of 7.34, a $PaCO_2$ of 60, and a HCO_3 of 32, he has a chronic respiratory acidosis with appropriate metabolic compensation. Clues to the chronic nature of his disease are the history (COPD), the higher HCO_3, and the near-normal pH. This patient is also speaking easily; someone who was previously normal would be stuporous or comatose with a $PaCO_2$ of 60.

Another case: A patient who received too much morphine is now stuporous. His ABG shows a pH of 7.26, a $PaCO_2$ of 55, and a HCO_3 of 27. He has a respiratory acidosis, and his expected HCO_3 is 26. Therefore, he has an acute respiratory acidosis with appropriate metabolic compensation.

Finally, consider an unconscious patient brought in from a house fire. His pH is 7.13, his $PaCO_2$ is 60, and his HCO_3 is 16. His primary problem is respiratory (you could call it metabolic and work it up from that angle—dealer's choice), and his expected HCO_3 is 26, which is higher than the measured HCO_3. He has a combined respiratory and metabolic acidosis. In this case, cyanide is the culprit.

In respiratory alkalosis, the same rules about acute and chronic conditions apply. Chronic respiratory alkalosis is usually due to pregnancy, chronic hypoxemia, chronic liver disease, and medication side effects.

Compensation for Respiratory Alkalosis:

- **Acute: HCO_3 drops 2 for every 10 the $PaCO_2$ falls**
- **Chronic: HCO_3 drops 5 for every 10 the $PaCO_2$ falls**

An example: A patient is brought in after sudden onset of dyspnea and tachypnea (30-34 breaths per minute). Her pH is 7.52, her $PaCO_2$ is 25, and her HCO_3 is 21. The expected HCO_3 is therefore 21 (by the above formula), so she has an <u>acute respiratory alkalosis with appropriate metabolic compensation</u>. CT scan shows a pulmonary embolism.

After you see that patient, you are asked to see an elderly lady who has been vomiting for two days. History reveals that she has accidentally been taking her theophylline three times a day instead of twice, and her theophylline level is 30 (toxic). Her ABG shows a pH of 7.58, a $PaCO_2$ of 30, and a HCO_3 of 29. She has a <u>chronic respiratory alkalosis</u> (a known side effect of theophylline, especially high doses) as well as a <u>metabolic alkalosis</u> from vomiting.

What about all of those formulas? Sorry, there are no shortcuts in Step Two. Either write them down in a notepad or memorize them. The more tech-savvy will keep them readily available on a smartphone. As you become more of an aficionado, the formulas will come to you easily.

Step Three: Mind the Gap

You'll remember that there are two types of metabolic acidosis—those that cause an anion gap, and those that don't. The anion gap, if you recall, is calculated as $[Na - (Cl + HCO_3)]$. The normal value is around 12, and accounts for unmeasured anions like plasma proteins. If the calculated gap is at least 3-4 higher than normal, consider it elevated. Hypoalbuminemia can falsely lower the anion gap, so the normal value should be the serum albumin multiplied by 3. Step Three of the method requires you to calculate the anion gap and create a differential diagnosis based on it. The differential can be remembered by the following mnemonics. Don't worry—remembering how to spell 'mnemonic' is harder than solving acid-base problems!

A Few Causes of an Elevated Anion Gap Acidosis (MUDPILES)

Methanol poisoning
Uremia
Diabetic ketoacidosis
Paraldehyde poisoning
Iron, Isoniazide poisoning
Lactic acidosis
Ethylene glycol poisoning, Ethanol-related ketoacidosis
Salicylate poisoning, Starvation ketoacidosis, Sepsis

A Few Causes of a Non-Anion Gap Acidosis (HARD UP)

Hyperchloremia (saline, TPN)
Addison's disease, Acetazolamide
Renal tubular acidosis
Diarrhea

Ureteral diversion procedures
Pancreatic problems (pseudocyst, fistula)

The presence or absence of an anion gap will help you determine the cause of a metabolic acidosis. Sometimes, it is the only clue that a metabolic acidosis exists. In addition, the rise in the anion gap above normal should correlate with the drop in HCO_3 from the normal value (24). If the HCO_3 is higher than expected, there is a coexisting metabolic alkalosis. If the HCO_3 is lower than expected, there may be a coexisting non-anion gap acidosis present.

Here's a case: A 23-year-old diabetic comes to the hospital in shock. His parents say that he has been vomiting constantly for 4 days. Your colleague asks you to help him decipher the patient's blood gas and chemistry. His blood glucose is 399, his serum Na is 133, the Cl is 90, and the HCO_3 is 20. His pH is 7.20 and the $PaCO_2$ is 40. What's going on?

1. The primary disorder is a metabolic acidosis, probably DKA (confirmed by elevated serum acetone).

2. The expected $PaCO_2$ should be 38, and his is 40—therefore, he has a metabolic acidosis with appropriate respiratory compensation.

3. His anion gap is 23—elevated, consistent with DKA. But wait! The rise in the anion gap is 11 (23-12), so his HCO_3 should have dropped by around 11 to give us a serum bicarbonate of 13 (24-11). His HCO_3 is 20, which is significantly higher than expected. This suggests a coexisting metabolic alkalosis, brought about by his vomiting and dehydration. The final word? This patient has diabetic ketoacidosis with a concomitant metabolic alkalosis due to volume depletion.

In closing....

Hopefully, this method will help you sort out the confusing acid-base problems you will come across in clinical practice. Remember that practice makes perfect—go through every step on every ABG you come across. You don't need to tell anyone how easy it is—in fact, you can mutter some things about "logarithmic changes" and "titratable acidity in the setting of the Isohydric Principle" while you easily solve the problem, if you want to make it look as hard as everyone else seems to think it is.

Infectious Disease

What To Know On Rounds

- Antibiotics the patient is receiving, and duration of therapy
- Culture and susceptibility results
- Presumed and known sources of infection
- Source control measures that either have been performed or need to be performed
- Therapeutic drug levels and monitoring for toxicity

What You Need To Survive

Infections and sepsis are seen in every type of ICU, either as a primary diagnosis or as a complication of critical illness. There's a reason why there are whole textbooks and an entire subspecialty devoted to treating infections—it's complicated! There's no way to cover all the ins and outs of infectious disease in this section, so we'll focus on what's commonly* seen in critical care. This section covers:

- Seven rules covering the basics of treating infections
- Steps you can take to prevent infections in the ICU
- Conditions that require definitive source control
- Guidelines for empiric coverage of common infections
- A table of antibiotic coverage for different organisms

---

* We won't even get into fungal infections, COVID, viral illnesses, or the weird infections found in burn and transplant units. This is definitely an area where you need to do some more reading if you want to get good at it.

103

Seven Rules for Treating Infections in the ICU

The first rule is that **all infections are local**. That is, the likely pathogens causing illness (and their susceptibility to different antibiotics) will vary depending on your region, your hospital, and even your unit. The *Pseudomonas aeruginosa* seen in a community-based hospital is going to have a much different resistance pattern than the *Pseudomonas* found in a burn unit. The differential diagnosis for an acute febrile respiratory illness includes Hantavirus in the American Southwest, but that infection would be considered a zebra[*] in Quebec. And the infections seen in transplant recipients are a whole separate issue. This book cannot possibly cover all the variation in the field of Infectious Disease. So, when you see the table for empiric coverage, that's based on typical academic and community hospitals in much of the United States. It's also based on infections bad enough to land the patient in ICU, so this obviously doesn't apply to outpatient care or even non-critical hospital admissions.

The second rule: empiric coverage should be broad and cover both the usual and the can't-miss pathogens.

The third rule: empiric coverage is fine at first, but the antibiotic regimen should be targeted at what's identified. Review your culture results (you *did* get cultures, right?) and narrow the coverage based on what you find.

The fourth rule: reconsider the need for antibiotics *every day*. This especially applies to patients with negative culture results who are improving. Fight the urge to continue antibiotics "just because"[†] and only treat proven or likely infections. A good rule of thumb is that you have three days for empiric antibiotics—after that, you either need a positive culture or a really good reason to continue.

---

[*] "When you hear hoofbeats, think horses, not zebras." So, the saying goes. Unless you're in Kenya, where zebras are much more common than horses—in that case, think zebras, not horses. Local.

[†] Antibiotic resistance is a major issue. It's not the broad-spectrum coverage given up front that causes the problems; rather, it's the prolonged duration of therapy that promotes resistance.

The fifth rule: every antibiotic has the potential for toxicity, even when dosed appropriately. Follow therapeutic levels and be sure to consider drug toxicity for any deterioration in a patient's condition.

The sixth rule: when you consider an infection, consider the host. Immunocompromised or debilitated patients get infections that immunocompetent, otherwise healthy patients don't.

The seventh rule: **never** pass up the opportunity to evacuate pus.[*] Infected pleural fluid, bile, and urine must be drained. Infected fascia must be debrided. Source control is a key part of the treatment of sepsis and cannot be deferred.

Infection Prevention in the ICU

- Your mother was right—**WASH YOUR HANDS!** Seriously. Wash them going into the room, and again coming out. Alcohol foam is fine most of the time. "Foam in, foam out."
- Remind other members of the team to wash their hands. Set the example and don't be afraid to say anything.
- If a patient has *C. difficile* or if you get anything visible on your hands, alcohol foam won't cut it. Good old soap and water to the rescue.[†]
- All ventilated patients need regular oral care.
- Elevate the head of the bed of ventilated patients to 30 degrees.
- Prep, drape, and use maximal barriers when placing central lines.
- Chlorhexidine and povidone iodine are great, but they have to dry before they're effective. Scrub the skin and then wait a few. Don't start until the skin is dry.
- Consider the need for indwelling lines and tubes *every day*. Not everyone in the ICU needs a Foley catheter (or a central line).

---

[*] Pus, poop, piss, and babies—they all have to come out.

[†] Seriously, THREE bullets on handwashing? Yes, seriously. For some reason we still don't do a good job with this. Hold yourself and others accountable.

Some Infections That Require Definitive Source Control

Abscess (superficial, deep, intraabdominal)	Drainage (either by incision or percutaneous drain)
Pleural empyema	Tube thoracostomy
Acute cholecystitis	Cholecystostomy Cholecystectomy (if necrotic or emphysematous)
Pyonephrosis	Percutaneous nephrostomy
Emphysematous pyelonephritis	Nephrectomy
Necrotizing fasciitis	Surgical debridement Hyperbaric oxygen therapy (as adjunct)
Line infections	Remove the line
Infective endocarditis	Surgery is indicated for infected prosthetic valves; fungal endocarditis; vegetations > 1 cm; cardiac conduction disturbances; and valvular insufficiency

Empiric Treatment for Common Infections

Source	Likely Pathogens	Coverage
Community-acquired Pneumonia	S. pneumoniae M. catarrhalis H. influenzae S. aureus (incl. MRSA) L. pneumophila	Ceftriaxone AND Azithromycin OR Doxycycline OR Levofloxacin, ± Vancomycin
Healthcare-associated Pneumonia (> 48 hours inpatient)	P. aeruginosa E. coli Enteric GNR MRSA	Vancomycin AND Piperacillin-tazobactam OR Cefepime OR Meropenem
Necrotizing Skin and Soft Tissue Infections*	Group A streptococci S. aureus (incl. MRSA) E. coli P. aeruginosa C. perfringens	Clindamycin AND Vancomycin AND [Ceftriaxone + Metronidazole] OR Piperacillin-tazobactam
Pyelonephritis†	E. coli P. mirabilis K. pneumoniae	Ceftriaxone OR Ciprofloxacin OR Cefepime
Bloodstream Infection	S. aureus (incl. MRSA) Group A streptococci E. coli Enteric GNR	Vancomycin AND Cefepime OR Piperacillin-tazobactam
Intra-abdominal Infections	E. coli Bacteroides spp. K. oxytoca	Piperacillin-tazobactam OR [Ceftriaxone + Metronidazole]
Meningitis	S. pneumoniae N. meningiditis H. influenzae L. monocytogenes	Ceftriaxone AND Vancomycin AND Ampicillin

---

* Urgent surgical consultation is mandatory!

† If a patient has a UTI bad enough to put him in the ICU, some sort of renal imaging is warranted (CT or ultrasound). Obstructions must be relieved and abscesses must be drained.

	GRAM POSITIVE COCCI				GRAM NEGATIVE RODS				ANAEROBES AND ATYPICALS			
	MRSA	MSSA	Streptococci	Enterococci	E. coli	Klebsiella	Enteric GNR	Pseudomonas	Oral Anaerobes	Bacteroides	Legionella	Rickettsia
Vancomycin	■	■	■	■					■			
Nafcillin		■	■									
Ampicillin-sulbactam		■	■	■	■	■	■		■	■		
Piperacillin-tazobactam		■	■	■	■	■	■	■	■	■		
Aztreonam					■	■	■	■				
Cefazolin		■	■		■	■						
Ceftriaxone		■	■		■	■	■					
Ceftazidime			■		■	■	■	■				
Cefepime		■	■		■	■	■	■				
Aminoglycosides					■	■	■	■				
Azithromycin		■	■								■	
Doxycycline			■				■				■	■
Ciprofloxacin					■	■	■	■			■	
Levofloxacin		■	■		■	■	■	■			■	
Ertapenem		■	■		■	■	■		■	■		
Meropenem		■	■		■	■	■	■	■	■		
Clindamycin	■	■	■						■			
Metronidazole									■	■		

Shaded = Generally Susceptible
Remember That All Infections Are Local!
Consult your ICU's antibiogram to make sure your coverage is adequate

Bleeding and Clotting

What You Need To Survive

Hematology is a broad field that either affects or is affected by many critical illnesses and injuries. The differential diagnosis and workup of anemia, neutropenia, and thrombocytopenia is extensive and beyond the scope of this book. We will focus on bleeding and clotting problems commonly encountered in the ICU. This section covers:

- DVT prophylaxis regimens
- Therapeutic anticoagulation
- Diagnosis of heparin-induced thrombocytopenia
- Massive transfusion protocols
- Using the thromboelastograph for the acutely bleeding patient
- Reversal of anticoagulation

DVT Prophylaxis

Virtually every patient in the ICU is moderate- or high-risk for deep venous thrombosis. Typical prophylaxis against this condition:

- Enoxaparin 40 mg SC daily
- Heparin 5000 units SC q8h for patients with a GFR < 30
- Enoxaparin 0.5 mg/kg q12h (especially for patients with a BMI over 40)

- Fondaparinux 2.5 mg SC daily (long-acting, but no risk of heparin-induced thrombocytopenia)

Consider monitoring anti-Xa levels, drawn 4 hours after dosing, for enoxaparin therapy (both prophylaxis and therapeutic anticoagulation).

Pharmacologic prophylaxis is superior to sequential compression devices (SCDs). The addition of SCDs to pharmacologic DVT prophylaxis doesn't appear to confer any benefit. SCDs should be used when there is a contraindication to pharmacologic therapy.

Therapeutic Anticoagulation

Agent	Dose	Monitoring*	Typical Indication
Low-intensity heparin	60 U/kg bolus, then 12 U/kg/hr	aPTT 40-60	Acute coronary syndrome
High-intensity heparin	80 U/kg bolus, then 18 U/kg/hr	aPTT 70-90	DVT, pulmonary embolism, ventricular thrombus
Enoxaparin	1 mg/kg SC q12h, or 1.5 mg/kg SC qd	Anti-Xa level 0.6-1.2 U/mL	DVT, pulmonary embolism, acute coronary syndrome, ventricular thrombus
Argatroban	2 mcg/kg/min to start, up to 10 mcg/kg/min	aPTT 1.5-3.0 times baseline	Heparin-induced thrombocytopenia
Fondaparinux	<50 kg: 5 mg SC daily 50-100 kg: 7.5 mg SC daily >100 kg: 10 mg SC daily	Anti-Xa level calibrated to fondaparinux; lab-specific	Heparin-induced thrombocytopenia, or patients with thrombosis at high risk for HIT

---

* This is all lab-dependent—your values may be different at your hospital.

110

4T Score for Heparin-Induced Thrombocytopenia

Parameter	0 points	1 point	2 points
Thrombocytopenia	Fall in platelets < 30% Lowest platelet count < 10K	Fall in platelets 30-50% Lowest platelet count 10-19K	Fall in platelets > 50% Lowest platelet count ≥ 20K
Timing	Fall in platelets <4 days, without recent exposure	Fall in platelets after 10 days Fall in platelets ≤ 1 day with exposure 30-100 days ago	Fall in platelets 5-10 days Fall in platelets ≤ 1 day with exposure within 30 days
Thrombosis	None	Progressive or recurrent thrombosis; non-necrotizing skin lesions	New thrombosis or skin necrosis; acute systemic reaction after IV heparin bolus
Other cause of thrombocytopenia	Definite	Possible	None

Scoring

≤ 3 points: low probability for HIT (< 5%)

4-5 points: intermediate probability for HIT (14%)

6-8 points: high probability for HIT (64%)

Consider testing for HIT (PF4 antibodies, ELISA, serotonin-release assay) and using non-heparin anticoagulation (argatroban, fondaparinux) for intermediate- and high-probability patients.

Massive Transfusion Protocols

Massive transfusion protocols (MTP) are designed to replicate whole blood transfusion, which has been proven to be superior to component-based therapy targeted toward laboratory endpoints. In other words, it's better to give FFP along with PRBC than to wait for the PT/INR to become abnormal.

Most trauma centers use a 1:1:1 MTP. This refers to the ratio of units of PRBC, plasma, and platelets transfused. A pooled plateletpheresis unit is the same as six units of platelets (the old "six pack"). So, a typical MTP would be 6 units PRBC, 6 units FFP, and one plateletpheresis unit. Additional transfusion should follow this ratio. For non-trauma patients (GI hemorrhage, obstetrical hemorrhage), a PRBC:FFP ratio of 2:1 seems to be just as effective and reduces the amount of plasma transfused; this may reduce the risk of TRALI and other complications. For simplicity's sake, it's reasonable to keep the PRBC: FFP ratio between 1:1 and 2:1.

Additional components of the MTP include cryoprecipitate (for fibrinogen replacement) and tranexamic acid (TXA) for antifibrinolytic activity. Calcium chloride or calcium gluconate should be administered empirically with MTP, as the citrate used in stored blood products chelates ionized calcium. Active rewarming and correction of acidosis are also essential.

The indication for MTP is ongoing hemorrhage. Once the bleeding has been controlled (in the OR, in the angiography suite, with banding of varices, etc.) it's reasonable to use laboratory endpoints to deescalate therapy. The thromboelastograph (TEG) is also helpful in this regard. Laboratory tests that should be obtained at the initiation of MTP and during the resuscitation include:

- CBC
- PT/INR, aPTT
- Fibrinogen level
- Type and crossmatch (initially the MTP will be uncrossmatched emergency release, but the blood bank will need to crossmatch blood products for ongoing transfusion)
- Ionized calcium (often available with the arterial blood gas)
- ABG
- Lactate
- Serum electrolytes
- Hepatic and renal function testing
- Thromboelastograph (if available)

Using the Thromboelastograph (TEG)

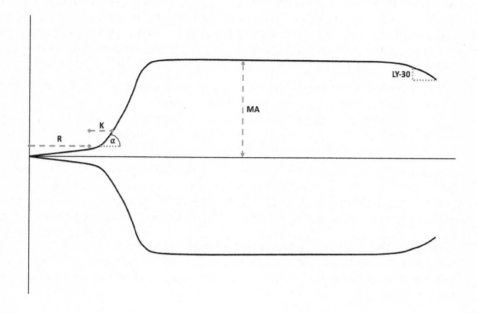

The TEG is a graphical representation of the clotting cascade. While it is not a substitute for other measures of coagulation (platelet count, PT/INR, aPTT), it does provide a better overview of the patient's coagulation status and can be a guide to transfusion therapy. The TEG can best be visualized by thinking of a filament inserted into a tube of blood. As the tube is spun, a clot forms around the filament.

TEG Parameters[*]

R-time: The R-time (reaction time) is the time it takes for the clot to go from 0 to 2 mm thick. This is driven by the intrinsic and extrinsic pathways of the clotting cascade and reflects the availability of clotting factor and the ability to form thrombin. The normal R-time is 5-10 minutes.

- R-time *lower* than normal: hypercoagulability; rapid thrombin generation in the setting of bleeding
- R-time *higher* than normal: deficiency of clotting factor; inhibition of clotting (heparin, thrombin inhibitors); consumptive coagulopathy

K-time: the K-time (kinetics time) is the time it takes for the clot to go from 2 to 20 mm thick. This is due to conversion of fibrinogen to fibrin, fibrin deposition, and cross-linking. It is also dependent, to a lesser extent, on platelet function. The normal K-time is 1-3 minutes.

α-angle: the α-angle is the angle between the end of the R-time and the rate of maximal clot formation. It corresponds closely with the K-time and is also driven primarily by fibrinogen. The normal α-angle is 53-73 degrees.

- K-time *lower* than normal, with α-angle *higher* than normal: hypercoagulability; rapid clot formation in the setting of hemorrhage
- K-time *higher* than normal, with α-angle *lower* than normal: fibrinogen depletion; consumptive coagulopathy; dysfibrinogenemia; significant platelet deficiency or dysfunction

MA: the MA (maximal amplitude) is the maximum thickness of the clot and is largely dependent on platelet function. The normal MA is 50-70 mm.

- MA *lower* than normal: thrombocytopenia; thrombasthenia; platelet inhibition with medications; uremic platelet dysfunction
- MA *higher* than normal: hypercoagulability

---

[*] The values and times may vary depending on what kind of TEG your lab runs, so always look at the normal values listed with your results. The Rapid-TEG, for example, has much shorter normal values.

LY-30: the LY-30 represents the percentage of clot that is lysed 30 minutes after reaching maximal amplitude. The normal LY-30 is 0-8%.

- LY-30 *higher* than normal: accelerated fibrinolysis; presence of activated plasminogen

The TEG is useful during massive transfusion; it is also helpful in treating patients who have coagulation derangements but who may not actually have a higher bleeding risk (cirrhotics, for example). The TEG does have some limitations. It does not indicate specific coagulation factor deficiencies or distinguish between intrinsic and extrinsic pathway problems, and as such it cannot entirely replace the conventional coagulation labs like aPTT, PT/INR, and fibrinogen level. The TEG also cannot be used to screen for DVT or PE. Most importantly, the R-time may be normal in the setting of warfarin therapy, even with a therapeutic INR.

Massive Transfusion Components

Blood Product or Adjunct	Typical Dose	Resuscitation Endpoint	TEG Parameter*
PRBC	1-4 units at a time	Hemoglobin > 8 g/dL	None
FFP	1-4 units at a time	INR < 1.5	R-time < 10 min
Platelets	1-2 pooled unit at a time	Platelet count > 50K/mcL	MA > 50 mm
Cryoprecipitate	5-10 units at a time	Fibrinogen > 150 mg/dL	K-time < 3 min α-angle > 53 degrees
TXA	1 g bolus, then 1 g infused over 8 hours	None	LY30 < 10%
Calcium	1 g calcium chloride, or 3 g calcium gluconate†	Ionized calcium > 1.10 mmol	

---

* This is for the standard TEG. The Rapid TEG or rotational thromboelastometry (ROTEM) may have different values. Consult your lab's reference range.

† Preferred for peripheral venous administration

Anticoagulation Reversal for Life-Threatening Hemorrhage*

Unfractionated Heparin and Low Molecular Weight Heparins

Medication	Reversal Agent	Dose
Heparin	Protamine	Immediate: 1-1.5 mg/100 units heparin 30-60 minutes after dose: 0.5-0.75 mg/100 units heparin > 60 minutes after dose: 0.25-0.5 mg/100 units heparin
Enoxaparin	Protamine[†]	< 8 hours after dose: 1 mg/1 mg enoxaparin 8-12 hours after dose: 0.5 mg/1 mg enoxaparin > 12 hours after dose: no reversal needed Maximum dose: 50 mg
Dalteparin	Protamine	1 mg protamine/100 units dalteparin Maximum dose: 50 mg
Fondaparinux	Factor VIIa aPCC (FEIBA)[‡]	90 mcg/kg (limited data) 50 U/kg (limited data)

---

* For abnormal lab values without bleeding, or minor bleeding, reversal may not be warranted.

† Protamine only reverses 60-75% of the anti-Xa activity of LMWH and can have anticoagulant activity itself!

‡ Activated prothrombin complex concentrate with Factor VIII inhibitor bypassing activity

117

Warfarin

Reversal Agent	Dose	Comments
Vitamin K	10 mg IV (not PO, IM, or SC)	Lowers INR in 1-2 hours
3-Factor PCC*	INR 2-4: 25 U/kg INR 4-6: 35 U/kg INR > 6: 50 U/kg	
4-Factor PCC†	INR 2-4: 25 U/kg INR 4-6: 35 U/kg INR > 6: 50 U/kg OR 1500 U (fixed dose)	
Fresh Frozen Plasma (FFP)	10-15 mL/kg (4-5 units in most adults)	FFP is 200-250 mL/unit Risk of transfusion reaction

---

* Prothrombin complex concentrate; trade name is Profilnine

† Trade name is Kcentra

118

Direct Oral Anticoagulants

Medication	Reversal Agent	Dose
Dabigatran[*]	Idarucizumab	5 g (recommended reversal agent)
	aPCC (FEIBA)	50 U/kg
	Cryoprecipitate	2 units if fibrinogen is < 200 mg/dL
Apixaban Rivaroxaban[†]	4-Factor PCC	25-50 U/kg (recommended reversal agent), maximum dose 5000 U.
	aPCC (FEIBA)	25 U/kg
	Andexanet	400 mg bolus, followed by 480 mg over 2 hours
Edoxaban Betrixaban[‡]	Unknown	There is limited or no data on reversal agents for these medications. Expert consultation is recommended.

Antiplatelet Medications

- DDAVP 0.4 mcg/kg IV (one dose) may reduce the antiplatelet activity of aspirin and clopidogrel by enhancing endothelial release of Von Willebrand Factor and Factor VIII.
- Platelet transfusion is commonly done (2-3 pooled units), but there is little evidence of effectiveness; in neurosurgical patients, this was associated with increased mortality in the PATCH trial.

---

[*] Trade name is Pradaxa; it is a direct thrombin (Factor IIa) inhibitor.

[†] Trade names, respectively, are Eliquis and Xarelto. They are Factor Xa inhibitors.

[‡] Trade names, respectively, are Savaysa and Bevyxxa. They are Factor Xa inhibitors.

Endocrine

What You Need To Survive

There are several endocrinologic disorders that can lead to ICU admission; additionally, uncontrolled diabetes mellitus and hyperglycemia are common in critical care. This section covers:

- Treatment of diabetic ketoacidosis and HHS
- Blood glucose management in critical care
- Treatment of adrenal insufficiency
- Treatment of central and nephrogenic diabetes insipidus
- Treatment of thyroid storm and myxedema coma

Diabetic ketoacidosis (DKA)

Diagnosis:

- Elevated blood glucose, particularly in the setting of Type 1 diabetes mellitus
- Elevated anion gap (Na^+ - Cl^- - HCO_3^-), typically > 16
- Evidence of ketosis—positive urine ketones, elevated serum ß-hydroxybutyrate

The pH is typically low in DKA, but it may be higher if there is concomitant intravascular volume depletion causing a contraction alkalosis. The low pH from DKA may be balanced out by the high pH of volume depletion. That's a good reason to always check the anion gap!

Common causes of DKA:
- Noncompliance with insulin regimen, or an improperly dosed insulin regimen (most common)
- Infection
- Pregnancy
- Myocardial ischemia
- Pancreatitis
- Trauma

Treatment of DKA:
1. Insulin is the mainstay of treatment. A bolus of 0.1 unit/kg may be given IV, but that isn't mandatory. An insulin infusion of 0.1. unit/kg/hour is necessary.
2. Volume depletion is typical in most patients with DKA and may be due to several factors. Hyperglycemia (glucose > 250) typically causes an osmotic diuresis and free water loss. Vomiting is common, particularly if the acidemia is severe. Poor oral intake is also common. The goal of treatment is to restore euvolemia.
   a. A 30-40 mL/kg bolus of isotonic fluid is a good starting point. Obviously, this is not always necessary and should be modified based on the patient's volume status (especially with renal and cardiac disease).
   b. Lactated Ringer's (LR) is preferred over 0.9% saline (NS), especially if the pH is < 7.1. The high chloride load with saline may exacerbate the acidosis.
   c. Following the fluid bolus, an infusion of 0.45% saline at 3-4 mL/kg/hour (200-250 mL/hr in most adults) will help restore euvolemia and correct for free water losses.
   d. Once the blood glucose is less than 250, change the IV fluid to D5-0.45% saline. The addition of dextrose lets you keep the insulin infusion going without causing hypoglycemia.
3. The insulin infusion should be maintained until the ketoacidosis is corrected—that is, until the anion gap has normalized. **The purpose of the insulin drip is to treat ketoacidosis, not hyperglycemia**.
4. As the patient rebuilds his depleted intracellular glycogen stores, three electrolytes will go down—K^+, Mg^{++}, and PO_4^-. Measure these frequently and aggressively replace any deficits.

5. Obtain a blood chemistry profile every 4-6 hours to follow the serum electrolytes, renal function, and the anion gap.
6. Once the ketoacidosis has resolved (e.g., the anion gap has normalized), administer long-acting insulin like glargine. If the patient's home dose is known, that can be given. If not, 0.5 units/kg is a typical dose. Reduce this if the patient is not eating (and continue the dextrose infusion until he is). 2-3 hours after the long-acting insulin has been given, the insulin drip can be stopped.

Mistakes in the treatment of DKA:

- Thinking that fluids alone can treat the condition. Hyperglycemia may respond to IV fluids, but ketoacidosis won't. You must use insulin.
- Stopping the insulin infusion because of the blood glucose instead of the anion gap.
- Trying to lower the serum potassium early on in the patient's course. The serum K^+ is usually elevated, but this is because of the low pH and not due to potassium excess. The serum K^+ will drop with the correction of the acidosis and due to insulin itself causing an intracellular shift.
- Keeping the patient NPO while the insulin drip is on. Once she starts feeling better, she'll be hungry. DKA is a starvation state and it doesn't make sense to starve a starving patient. Let her eat.
- Giving regular (short-acting) insulin instead of long-acting insulin before turning off the insulin drip. If you give short-acting insulin it'll be gone in 3-6 hours. Then the patient will go back into DKA.

Hyperglycemic Hyperosmolar Syndrome

Hyperglycemic Hyperosmolar Syndrome (HHS) is more common in Type 2 diabetics. It differs from DKA in that the serum ketones aren't as elevated (but still can be—it's a misnomer to call this state "nonketotic," since there is an element of starvation present). The serum sodium is also considerably more elevated in HHS, leading to the hyperosmolar state.

The precipitating factors are similar to those seen with DKA. Infection, myocardial ischemia, and pancreatitis are very common causes.

The treatment of HHS is likewise similar to the treatment of DKA, but there are a few differences that need to be considered:

- The volume depletion seen in HHS is usually more profound. If most DKA patients are 3-4 liters down, most HHS patients are 8-10 liters down.
- The hypernatremia will require more free water replacement. However, this isn't as much of a priority as correcting hypovolemia.
- An insulin infusion should be started at 0.1 units/kg/hour, like with DKA, but the blood glucose is the target for treatment and not the anion gap (since there isn't significant ketoacidosis). Try to lower the blood glucose by 100-200 mg/dL per hour.
- Since HHS is typically secondary to a systemic illness and not simply noncompliance, be sure to investigate for the precipitating cause.

Treatment of Hyperglycemia in the ICU

Many patients in the ICU will become hyperglycemic, even if they don't have diabetes mellitus. This typically needs to be treated with a combination of long-acting insulin (like glargine) and a sliding scale correction with regular insulin. A typical starting insulin order looks like this:

1. Insulin glargine 0.1 units/kg subcutaneous QPM
2. Measure point-of-care blood glucose Q6H
3. Sliding scale correction based on blood glucose (mg/dL)
   a. 150-200: 2 units regular insulin IV
   b. 201-150: 4 units regular insulin IV
   c. 251-300: 6 units regular insulin IV
   d. 301-350: 8 units regular insulin IV
   e. 351-400: 10 units regular insulin IV
   f. > 400: notify treating team

Most hospitals will have a prewritten sliding scale correction protocol that can be ordered. Usually, it will also have different ranges for insulin-sensitive and insulin-resistant patients. The long-acting insulin can be adjusted by taking the amount of correction insulin needed in the last 24 hours, dividing that by 2, and then adding it to the long-acting dose. For example, a patient receiving 10 units of insulin glargine requires 16 units of correction over the last 24 hours. The insulin glargine dose should be increased by 8 units to 18.

In the early aughts, it became commonplace in critical care units to pursue a strategy of "tight" glycemic control. This targeted a blood glucose of 80-110 mg/dL rather than the more permissive strategy of 140-180 mg/dL. The purported benefits of tight glycemic control included fewer infections and better wound healing. Unfortunately, hypoglycemic events (leading to patient harm) became more common with this approach as well. Several large prospective randomized trials (Glucontrol and VISEP 2008; NICE-SUGAR 2009) have failed to show any benefit to tight glycemic control.

At the time of writing, a more moderate approach of keeping the blood glucose less than 180-200 seems to be the way to go. Most of the time this can be done with the combination of long- and short-acting insulin described above. However, there are times when an insulin infusion is needed.

Times when an insulin infusion may be necessary:
- Hyperglycemia that can't be treated effectively with subcutaneous insulin
- Surgical patients who require frequent trips to the OR, meaning they are kept NPO for prolonged periods of time
- Cardiac surgery (there is some evidence that tight glycemic control may prevent complications in this group of patients)
- Total parenteral nutrition (it's difficult to control the blood glucose with long-acting insulin when using TPN)

Adrenal Insufficiency

Adrenal insufficiency can be either primary or secondary. Primary adrenal insufficiency can be due to autoimmune suppression of adrenal gland function (Addison's disease); infections like tuberculosis or meningococcemia (which can cause bilateral adrenal hemorrhage); congenital disorders; malignancy; and surgical removal of the adrenal gland(s). Primary adrenal insufficiency affects both mineralocorticoid and glucocorticoid function.

Primary adrenal insufficiency (adrenal crisis) is often associated with electrolyte and metabolic disturbances:
- Hyponatremia
- Hypoglycemia
- Hypothermia
- Hypotension

- Hyperkalemia
- Hypercalcemia

The diagnosis can be made by checking a random cortisol level (typically < 5 mg/dL). An ACTH stimulation test can be done if the diagnosis is questionable.

Treatment of an adrenal crisis:

1. Immediate steroid administration
   a. Hydrocortisone 100 mg IV q8h
   b. If an ACTH stimulation test is needed, give dexamethasone 10 mg IV (one dose). This will support the patient and not compromise the test.
2. IV fluids with dextrose to treat hypotension and hypoglycemia
3. Correction of electrolyte abnormalities

Secondary adrenal insufficiency can occur in the setting of sepsis, high levels of circulating proinflammatory cytokines, and disorders involving the hypothalamic-pituitary-adrenal axis (pituitary tumors and hemorrhage, cerebral anoxia). Chronic glucocorticoid administration, leading to downregulation of endogenous cortisol release, is a common reason for secondary adrenal insufficiency.

Steroids are an ongoing controversy in critical care medicine, particularly in septic shock. The concept of "relative adrenal insufficiency" is that the adrenal glands are exhausted and unable to produce enough cortisol and endogenous catecholamines to maintain homeostasis. Numerous clinical trials have examined the benefit of using stress-dose steroids in septic shock, and there are strong opinions on both sides of the issue. It's become more of a matter of belief than evidence for some clinicians, which is decidedly unscientific.

Here's what we know, at the time of writing, about the clinical benefit of steroids in septic shock:

- There is no clear mortality benefit. Some trials have shown a 28-day mortality benefit, but by 90 days it seems to be a wash.
- Steroids do seem to help with refractory hypotension and do help lower the dose of norepinephrine needed to keep the MAP > 65.
- Some claim that steroids get patients out of the ICU sooner, but this is likely due to the abovementioned point that they help reduce the need for vasopressors and most hospitals require all patients on vasopressors to be in the ICU.

- On the other side, the adverse consequences of steroid administration do not seem to be as pronounced as previously believed. In the largest trials examining the issue, the rates of delirium, secondary infections, and bowel ischemia were not significantly higher in the patients receiving hydrocortisone. There was a higher incidence of hyperglycemia, as expected, but this can be easily treated.
- An ACTH stimulation test isn't necessary in most patients. It can be helpful if there are relative contraindications to steroid administration or if there is suspicion of primary adrenal insufficiency.
  - Check a baseline cortisol level
  - Administer 250 mcg of ACTH IV
  - Check cortisol levels at 30 and 60 minutes
  - An increase in the cortisol level by at least 9 mg/dL indicates preserved adrenal function
- The usual dose of stress-dose hydrocortisone for septic shock is 200-300 mg per day. This can be done by continuous infusion or in divided doses (50 mg q6h, 100 mg q8h).
- Fludrocortisone 50 mcg PO daily can be added to the hydrocortisone if there is a concern for mineralocorticoid deficiency (particularly with primary adrenal insufficiency).

Diabetes Insipidus

Diabetes insipidus (DI) can be central (absent production of antidiuretic hormone in the posterior pituitary gland) or nephrogenic (insensitivity to ADH in the collecting ducts of the nephron).

Central DI is most commonly seen with cerebral anoxia, but can also be seen with pituitary hemorrhage, trauma, and following neurosurgical procedures. It is characterized by hypernatremia and polyuria (often > 500-1000 mL of urine per hour). Urine osmolality is low, typically 50-150 mOsm/L.

Treatment of central DI:

1. Vasopressin (ADH)
   a. DDAVP 1 mcg IV q6h, OR
   b. Vasopressin 0.02 U/min
   c. DDAVP and Vasopressin can be increased as needed. Vasopressin infusion is preferred, as it can be titrated more quickly.

2. Isotonic fluids (Lactated Ringer's preferred) to maintain euvolemia—typically start at 100-150 mL/hr
3. Replace all urinary losses *in excess of 200 mL/hr* with D5W
   a. As an example: if a patient has 350 mL urine output over the last hour, 150 mL of D5W would be given. If the urine output is 200 mL in the next hour, no D5W is given.
4. Follow serum sodium levels q4-6h
5. Goals of treatment
   a. Urine output 50-200 mL/hr
   b. Fall in serum sodium by 1-3 mEq per hour
   c. Hold DDAVP or Vasopressin for urine output < 50 mL/hr, or serum sodium < 140 mEq/L

Nephrogenic DI is typically due to medication toxicity (lithium, especially) and can also be seen with polycystic kidney disease and other disorders. The hypernatremia and polyuria is not as pronounced as it is with central DI. The urine osmolality is lower than the serum (indicating a lack of free water reabsorption in the setting of hypernatremia).

Treatment of nephrogenic DI:

- Free water supplementation with D5W or enteral water flushes
- Thiazide diuretics limit free water excretion in the distal convoluted tubule. Although it seems counterintuitive to give diuretics in the setting of polyuria, it increases urine osmolarity and limits free water losses, paradoxically reducing the urine output.

Thyrotoxicosis and Thyroid Storm

Thyrotoxicosis and thyroid storm can occur primarily, or in response to stress (infections, surgery). The TSH is very low and free T3/T4 levels are elevated.

Clinical features:

- Tachydysrhythmias
- Hyperthermia
- Elevated LFTs
- Malignant hypertension
- CNS changes, particularly agitation (this is what separates thyrotoxicosis from thyroid storm)
- Proptosis and an enlarged, tender thyroid gland are often seen with Grave's disease, but the lack of these does not rule out the diagnosis

Treatment of Thyrotoxicosis and Thyroid Storm:

1. Control adrenergic tone with beta-blockade
   a. Esmolol infusion, 25-200 mcg/kg/min
   b. Propranolol 20-40 mg PO q6h (start this when enteral access is established, and wean off the esmolol as tolerated)
   c. Propranolol also helps prevent conversion of T4 to T3, which is why it's the preferred oral beta-blocker
2. Control hyperthermia
   a. Cooling blankets
   b. Acetaminophen
   c. Avoid aspirin—it can accelerate conversion of T4 to T3
3. Block thyroid hormone synthesis
   a. Propylthiouracil (PTU) 500-1000 mg PO, followed by 250 mg PO q4h
   b. Methimazole (MMI) can also be used but isn't as effective as PTU in the first 24 hours
4. Reduce the release of thyroid hormone
   a. Saturated solution of potassium iodide (SSKI) 5 drops PO q6 hours
   b. Do not give SSKI until an hour after the PTU has been given
5. Treat concomitant adrenal insufficiency
   a. Hydrocortisone 100 mg IV q8h
   b. Do not do an ACTH stimulation test first—treat empirically

Myxedema Coma

Myxedema coma (which doesn't always cause a coma) is severe hypothyroidism. This is often precipitated by myocardial ischemia, infection, surgery, or another stressful condition. The TSH is typically very elevated, with low T3/T4 levels.

Clinical Features:

- Bradycardia
- Hypotension
- Hypoglycemia
- Hypothermia
- CNS depression

Treatment of Myxedema:

1. Levothyroxine (synthetic T4) 300-500 mcg IV, then 50-100 mcg IV daily. Use lower doses in patients with cardiac disease.
2. Triiodothyronine (synthetic T3) 5-20 mcg IV, followed by 2.5-10 mcg IV q8h when the patient is in shock or markedly hypothermic. Use lower doses in older patients and those with cardiac risk factors or known cardiac disease.
3. Treat concomitant adrenal insufficiency
   a. Hydrocortisone 100 mg IV q8h
   b. Do not do an ACTH stimulation test first—treat empirically
   c. This is not a typo—hydrocortisone should be given for both myxedema and thyroid storm!

Nutritional Support

What To Know On Rounds

- Enteral feeding route and status
- Goal rate of tube feeding
- Water intake (may need adjustment based on sodium level)
- Results of metabolic cart study and nitrogen balance
- TPN necessity and planned duration of therapy

What You Need To Survive

The acute phase of critical injury or illness is associated with inflammation, increased glycogenolysis, hepatic gluconeogenesis, and insulin resistance. It is also associated with loss of skeletal muscle and very high rates of energy expenditure. Nutritional support is essential for critical patients. This section covers:

- Enteral nutrition initiation
- Nutritional goals for most patients
- Targeted nutritional therapy
- TPN composition

Initiation of Enteral Nutrition

Early enteral nutrition accomplishes two things—it provides some calories, including protein (less important), and helps prevent gut mucosal atrophy (more important, as this can lead to bacterial translocation and release of proinflammatory cytokines).

The ideal target for caloric intake has not been defined, and in many ways, this is an impossible task. There is too much variability in underlying patient health, comorbidities, and the nature of the critical condition itself for a precise recommendation to be made.

When NOT to feed:

- Bowel perforation or discontinuity
- Severe uncontrolled shock (high doses of multiple vasopressors, ongoing fluid/blood resuscitation)
- Active GI hemorrhage

In most other cases, enteral nutrition should be started within 24-48 hours of ICU admission. For patients who are unable to eat, feeding via a nasogastric tube is the preferred method. Nasoduodenal and nasojejunal tubes (aka Dobhoff tubes, small-bore feeding tubes, post- pyloric tubes, or "the yellow tube") can be placed if there is gastric dysmotility or an expectation of prolonged (3-6 weeks) artificial feeding. Contrary to popular belief, the rate of aspiration pneumonitis is no higher with NG tubes when compared with post-pyloric feeding. Patients who have had gastric bypass or other proximal GI tract surgery should have the post-pyloric tube placed under fluoroscopy.

Trophic feeding (10 mL/hr) is as good as full support, at least within the first week of critical illness, and may be preferable if the patient is in shock. Hypocaloric feeding (70% of estimated requirements) is preferable to overfeeding. The malnutrition seen in critical illness is not typically due to caloric deprivation; it seems to be more related to systemic inflammation, proinflammatory cytokines, and dysfunctional cellular use of nutrients.

General Nutritional Goals

- 25 kcal/kg/day of a commercially available formula
- Supplemental water flushes to provide a total fluid intake of 25-30 mL/kg/day
- 1.2-1.5 grams of protein/kg/day
- For weight-based feeding:
  - BMI < 18.5 kg/m^2: use the actual body weight (ABW)
  - BMI 18.5-29.9 kg/m^2: use the ABW
  - BMI ≥ 30 kg/m^2: calculate the predicted body weight (PBW) just like for vent settings. Then, calculate the adjusted body weight for caloric intake: *Adjusted Weight = PBW + 0.25(ABW - PBW)*

Most of the time, a simple approach toward enteral nutrition is sufficient. Targeted nutritional therapy may be helpful in patients who have undergone major surgery, prolonged respiratory failure, or other conditions leading to significant muscle loss.

Targeted Nutritional Therapy

The target for enteral nutrition has traditionally been determined using an equation like the revised Harris-Benedict.[*] The basal metabolic rate (BMR) is calculated, and then multiplied by a factor based on the type of illness or injury to provide a caloric goal.

Men:
BMR = (10 × weight in kg) + (6.25 × height in cm) − (5 × age in years) + 5

Women:
BMR = (10 × weight in kg) + (6.25 × height in cm) − (5 × age in years) − 161

Obviously, equations like this one (and the nearly 200 others that have been published) are a pain to calculate and don't consider any individual patient factors other than height, weight, age, and gender.

Metabolic Cart Study

A much more accurate method for determining the BMR, also known as the resting energy expenditure (REE), is indirect calorimetry using a metabolic cart. With this device, the patient's oxygen consumption (VO_2) and carbon dioxide production (VCO_2) are directly measured and used to calculate the REE and the respiratory quotient (RQ).

The RQ is the ratio of VCO_2 to VO_2 and reflects the balance of nutrient intake; it can also be used in critically ill patients as a measure of under- or overfeeding.

The daily caloric intake should be adjusted to provide the REE plus 300-500 kcal of nonprotein calories per day. The carbohydrate intake can be adjusted to keep the RQ < 0.95.

---

[*] First published in 1919, now over 100 years old; the Mifflin-St. Jeor revision was published in 1990.

Nitrogen Balance

The urine urea nitrogen can be measured using a 6- or 24-hour fluid collection. Use this to calculate the patient's nitrogen balance:

- 24 hour urine urea nitrogen (multiply by 4 if you do a 6-hour collection), PLUS
- 2 grams N to account for unmeasured skin losses, PLUS
- 2 grams N to account for unmeasured stool losses

Since protein is 16% elemental nitrogen, multiply the figure you just calculated by 6.25. That gives you the minimum amount of daily protein needed to prevent skeletal muscle catabolism. Ideally, you'll provide *more* than the minimum. This is called keeping the patient in a "positive nitrogen balance."

If the patient is septic, has chronic wounds, or has burn injuries, it may be difficult to keep him in a positive nitrogen balance no matter how much protein you provide.

Total Parenteral Nutrition (TPN)

TPN is necessary when a critically ill patient is anticipated to be unable to receive adequate enteral nutrition for at least 5-7 days. Common reasons for TPN include extensive bowel surgery, prolonged ileus, and enterocutaneous fistula. It's also helpful when the patient can receive enteral nutrition but when it's unlikely to be sufficient to meet his caloric needs for an extended period of time.

TPN requires the patient to have a central line and there is an increased risk of infection and encephalopathy. If TPN is going to be used for a prolonged period, a peripherally inserted central catheter (PICC) is desirable. If TPN is needed for more than a month, a tunneled catheter is preferred.

There are different commercially available solutions used to compound TPN, so you'll need to work with your ICU's nutritional specialist and pharmacist to provide it. A general TPN prescription provides:

- Energy: 25 kcal/kg/day
- Protein: 1-1.5 g/kg/day
- Lipids: 1 g/kg/day (adjusted if the patient is receiving propofol)
- Carbohydrates: 4 g/kg/day

- Water: 25-30 mL/kg/day
- Standard electrolytes (daily electrolytes, including Mg and PO_4, should be monitored)
- Trace elements and a multivitamin

Useful Sources of Information

I sincerely hope you've found *The ICU Survival Book* to be useful, but I'd be lying if I said it was the only thing you need to read to be a successful clinician in the ICU. Here are some resources that I find to be particularly good.

BOOKS

The ICU Book, by Paul Marino

This is widely regarded as one of the best books on critical care medicine (and acute care medicine in general). It's now in its fourth edition and is just as good as it was when I bought my first copy in 1999.

Procedures, Techniques, and Minimally Invasive Monitoring in Intensive Care Medicine, by Irwin, Rippe, Lisbon, and Heard

This excellent resource covers procedures that are commonly done in the ICU. Where it shines is in the discussion of clinical management—it doesn't just tell you *how* to do a procedure; it also teaches you *when* to do it.

Critical Care Physiology, by Robert Bartlett

This was published in 1995 but it's amazing how ahead of its time it is—prone positioning and low tidal volume ventilation is discussed *years* before they were considered standard treatments. Physiology doesn't change and this book is one of my favorites.

The Ventilator Book, by William Owens[*]

I may be biased but I wrote the book as a guide for people who don't do critical care medicine for a living. That includes students, nurses, residents, and APPs. If you want to learn more about that mysterious box called "the vent," pick up the most recent edition of TVB.

WEBSITES

onepagericu.com

If you thought the sections in this book were too long, Nick Mark has come up with some great one-page references to different aspects of critical care.

heart-lung.org

Jon-Emile Kenny has a collection of excellent writings and videos on his website that take a deep dive into the physiology and pathophysiology encountered in acute care medicine. These are well worth your time.

pulmccm.org

There's a lot of good information here, including reviews of recent clinical trials. For my money, however, the best part is the "ICU Physiology in 1000 Words" series, written by Jon-Emile Kenny.

emcrit.org/ibcc/toc

Josh Farkas has a continually updated Internet Book of Critical Care that examines many aspects of intensive care medicine. He also has a podcast that's worth checking out.

statusiatrogenicus.blogspot.com

Do you like challenging dogma and questioning conventional wisdom? Me too! Scott Aberegg has a real talent for it and has some excellent posts. You'll definitely learn a lot about statistics.

---

[*] Who?

About the Author

William Owens, MD, is the Director of the Medical Intensive Care Unit at Prisma Health Richland, a tertiary referral center in Columbia, SC, and a Clinical Associate Professor of Medicine with the University of South Carolina. He has also served on the faculty at the University of Pittsburgh School of Medicine.

Dr. Owens is a graduate of The Citadel and the University of South Carolina School of Medicine. He trained in Emergency Medicine at the Earl K. Long Medical Center in Baton Rouge, LA, which was followed by fellowship training in Critical Care Medicine at the University of South Florida in Tampa, FL. He is board-certified in Emergency Medicine and Critical Care Medicine. He has spoken at regional and national conferences and has published articles in the peer-reviewed medical literature. He has also authored three editions of *The Ventilator Book*, *The Advanced Ventilator Book*, and created The Ventilator App.

Throughout his career, Dr. Owens has been an active clinician and educator. He enjoys training physicians, nurses, and respiratory therapists in the care of the most seriously ill and injured patients and is a firm subscriber to a holistic approach to critical care medicine. He believes in the rational application of physiology and in always questioning our assumptions. He also has a strong professional and recreational interest in Wilderness Medicine.

Dr. Owens lives in Columbia, SC, with his wife and family—one college student and two high-schoolers. Other members of the household are a St. Bernard named Juliet and a beehive with about 60,000 bees. He enjoys mountain biking, whitewater kayaking, coaching lacrosse, and going on family adventures.

141

tension pneumothorax, 29, 31, 32

therapeutic anticoagulation, 110

thermodilution, 25

thromboelastograph, 112, 113

thyrotoxicosis and thyroid storm, 129

tidal volume, 45, 56, 57

Torsades de Pointes. See polymorphic ventricular tachycardia

total parenteral nutrition, 134

TPN. See total parenteral nutrition

transcutaneous pacing, 39

trophic feeding, 132

urine urea nitrogen, 134

vasodilatory shock, 16

vasopressin, 20, 127, 128

ventilator settings, 49

ventilator troubleshooting, 59

ventricular tachycardia, 37

ventriculostomy, 74, 77

Made in United States
North Haven, CT
01 May 2023

36099706R10093